ORTHOPEDIC CLINICS OF NORTH AMERICA

www.orthopedic.theclinics.com

Reconstruction

January 2020 • Volume 51 • Number 1

Editor-in-Chief

FREDERICK M. AZAR

ELSEVIER

1600 John F. Kennedy Boulevard ● Suite 1800 ● Philadelphia, Pennsylvania, 19103-2899.

http://www.orthopedic.theclinics.com

ORTHOPEDIC CLINICS OF NORTH AMERICA Volume 51, Number 1
January 2020 ISSN 0030-5898, ISBN-13: 978-0-323-75424-8

Editor: Lauren Boyle
Developmental Editor: Kristen Helm

Photocopying

Single photocopies of single articles may be made for personal use as allowed by national copyright laws. Permission of the Publisher and payment of a fee is required for all other photocopying, including multiple or systematic copying, copying for advertising or promotional purposes, resale, and all forms of document delivery. Special rates are available for educational institutions that wish to make photocopies for non-profit educational classroom use. For information on how to seek permission visit www.elsevier.com/permissions or call: (+44) 1865 843830 (UK)/(+1) 215 239 3804 (USA).

Derivative Works

Subscribers may reproduce tables of contents or prepare lists of articles including abstracts for internal circulation within their institutions. Permission of the Publisher is required for resale or distribution outside the institution. Permission of the Publisher is required for all other derivative works, including compilations and translations (please consult www.elsevier.com/permissions).

Electronic Storage or Usage

Permission of the Publisher is required to store or use electronically any material contained in this periodical, including any article or part of an article (please consult www.elsevier.com/permissions). Except as outlined above, no part of this publication may be reproduced, stored in a retrieval system or transmitted in any form or by any means, electronic, mechanical, photocopying, recording or otherwise, without prior written permission of the Publisher.

Notice

No responsibility is assumed by the Publisher for any injury and/or damage to persons or property as a matter of products liability, negligence or otherwise, or from any use or operation of any methods, products, instructions or ideas contained in the material herein. Because of rapid advances in the medical sciences, in particular, independent verification of diagnoses and drug dosages should be made.

Although all advertising material is expected to conform to ethical (medical) standards, inclusion in this publication does not constitute a guarantee or endorsement of the quality or value of such product or of the claims made of it by its manufacturer.

Orthopedic Clinics of North America (ISSN 0030-5898) is published quarterly by Elsevier Inc., 360 Park Avenue South, New York, NY 10010-1710. Months of issue are January, April, July, and October. Business and Editorial Offices: 1600 John F. Kennedy Blvd., Suite 1800, Philadelphia, PA 19103-2899. Customer Service Office: 3251 Riverport Lane, Maryland Heights, MO 63043. Periodicals postage paid at New York, NY and additional mailing offices. Subscription prices are $344.00 per year for (US individuals), $786.00 per year for (US institutions), $403.00 per year (Canadian individuals), $960.00 per year (Canadian institutions), $471.00 per year (international individuals), $960.00 per year (international institutions), $100.00 per year (US students), $100.00 per year for (Canadian students), $220.00 per year for (international students). Foreign air speed delivery is included in all *Clinics* subscription prices. All prices are subject to change without notice. **POSTMASTER:** Send change of address to *Orthopedic Clinics of North America*, **Elsevier Health Sciences Division, Subscription Customer Service, 3251 Riverport Lane, Maryland Heights, MO 63043. Customer Service (orders, claims, online, change of address): Elsevier Health Sciences Division, Subscription Customer Service, 3251 Riverport Lane, Maryland Heights, MO 63043. Tel: 1-800-654-2452 (U.S. and Canada); 314-447-8871 (outside U.S. and Canada). Fax: 314-447-8029. E-mail:** journalscustomerservice-usa@elsevier.com **(for print support);** journalsonlinesupport-usa@elsevier.com **(for online support).**

Reprints. For copies of 100 or more, of articles in this publication, please contact the Commercial Reprints Department, Elsevier Inc., 360 Park Avenue South, New York, NY 10010-1710. Tel.: 212-633-3874; Fax: 212-633-3820; E-mail: reprints@elsevier.com.

Orthopedic Clinics of North America is covered in *MEDLINE/PubMed* (*Index Medicus*), *Cinahl, Excerpta Medica,* and *Cumulative Index to Nursing and Allied Health Literature.*

EDITORIAL BOARD

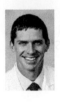

CONTRIBUTORS

AUTHORS

MELISSA M. ALLEN, MD, MSCR
Fellow, Pediatric Orthopedic Surgery, Baylor
College of Medicine, Houston, Texas, USA

MARK BAGG, MD
Hand Center of San Antonio, San Antonio,
Texas, USA

SOPHIA R. BAHAD
The Orthopedic Institute of North Texas, P.A.,
Frisco, Texas, USA

J. MICHAEL BENNETT, MD
Fondren Orthopaedic Group, Houston, Texas,
USA

CRISTIAN S. BORGES, MD
Member of the Brazilian Society for Surgery of
the Hand, Member of the Hand and
Microsurgery Division of the Orthopedics and
Traumatology Department, Santa Casa
Hospital Complex, Porto Alegre, Brazil;
Clinica da Mao ao Cotovelo, Porto Alegre, Rio
Grande do Sul, Brazil

PETER N. CHALMERS, MD
Assistant Professor, Department of
Orthopaedic Surgery, University of Utah
Medical Center, Salt Lake City, Utah, USA

STEPHEN CHAMBERS, MD
PGY-4 Resident, Department of Orthopaedic
Surgery and Biomedical Engineering,
University of Tennessee-Campbell Clinic,
Memphis, Tennessee, USA

MATTHEW S. CONTI, MD
Orthopaedic Surgery Resident, Hospital for
Special Surgery, New York, New York, USA

GREGORY D. DABOV, MD
Assistant Professor, Department of
Orthopaedic Surgery and Biomedical
Engineering, University of Tennessee-
Campbell Clinic, Memphis, Tennessee, USA

HUSSEIN A. ELKOUSY, MD
Fondren Orthopaedic Group, TERFSES
Shoulder and Elbow Fellowship, Texas
Orthopedic Hospital, Houston, Texas, USA

SCOTT J. ELLIS, MD
Associate Attending, Department of
Orthopaedic Foot and Ankle Surgery, Hospital
for Special Surgery, New York, New York, USA

MARCUS C. FORD, MD
Instructor, Department of Orthopaedic
Surgery and Biomedical Engineering,
University of Tennessee-Campbell Clinic,
Memphis, Tennessee, USA

JONATHAN H. GARFINKEL, MD
Orthopaedic Surgery Resident, Cedars-Sinai
Medical Center, Los Angeles, California, USA

TIMOTHY KAHN, MD
Orthopaedic Resident, Department of
Orthopaedic Surgery, University of Utah
Medical Center, Salt Lake City, Utah, USA

JUSTIN M. KANE, MD
Orthopaedic Surgeon, Foot and Ankle
Surgery Division, The Orthopedic Institute of
North Texas, P.A., Frisco, Texas, USA;
Professor of Surgery, Orthopaedics, Texas
A&M University Health Science Center,
College of Medicine, Bryan, Texas, USA

MADHAV A. KARUNAKAR, MD
Professor, Department of Orthopaedic
Surgery, Carolinas Medical Center, Atrium
Health Musculoskeletal Institute, Charlotte,
North Carolina, USA

ANITA KERKHOF, MS
Research Coordinator, Department of
Orthopaedic Surgery and Biomedical
Engineering, University of Tennessee-
Campbell Clinic, Memphis, Tennessee,
USA

CASEY J. KISER, MD
Fondren Orthopaedic Group, TERFSES
Shoulder and Elbow Fellowship, Texas
Orthopedic Hospital, Houston, Texas, USA

THEODORE T. MANSON, MD, MS
Associate Professor, Department of
Orthopaedic Surgery, R Adams
Cowley Shock Trauma Center, Baltimore,
Maryland, USA

ANTHONY M. MASCIOLI, MD
Assistant Professor, Department of
Orthopaedic Surgery and Biomedical
Engineering, University of
Tennessee-Campbell Clinic, Memphis,
Tennessee, USA

THOMAS L. MEHLHOFF, MD
Fondren Orthopaedic Group,
TERFSES Shoulder and Elbow Fellowship,
Texas Orthopedic Hospital, Houston, Texas,
USA

WILLIAM M. MIHALKO, MD, PhD
Professor, Department of Orthopaedic
Surgery and Biomedical Engineering,
University of Tennessee-Campbell Clinic,
Memphis, Tennessee, USA

BRENT J. MORRIS, MD
Fondren Orthopaedic Group, TERFSES
Shoulder and Elbow Fellowship, Texas
Orthopedic Hospital, Houston, Texas, USA

RYAN P. MULLIGAN, MD
Resident, Department of Orthopaedic Surgery
and Biomedical Engineering, University of
Tennessee-Campbell Clinic, Memphis,
Tennessee, USA

IAN MULLIKIN, MD
Hand Center of San Antonio, San Antonio,
Texas, USA

CRYSTAL A. PERKINS, MD
Children's Healthcare of Atlanta, Atlanta,
Georgia, USA

MILTON B. PIGNATARO, MD
Member of the Brazilian Society for Surgery of
the Hand, Chief of the Hand and Microsurgery
Division of the Orthopedics and Traumatology

Department, Santa Casa Hospital Complex,
Porto Alegre, Brazil; Clinica da Mao ao
Cotovelo, Porto Alegre, Rio Grande do Sul,
Brazil

OLIVIA M. RICE, MD
Resident, Department of Orthopaedic
Surgery, Carolinas Medical Center, Atrium
Health Musculoskeletal Institute, Charlotte,
North Carolina, USA

SCOTT B. ROSENFELD, MD
Associate Professor of Orthopaedic
Surgery, Baylor College of Medicine,
Associate Chief of Research and Education,
Director of the Hip Preservation Center,
Texas Children's Hospital, Houston, Texas,
USA

PAULO H. RUSCHEL, MD
Member of the Brazilian Society for Surgery of
the Hand, Member of the Hand and
Microsurgery Division of the Orthopedics and
Traumatology Department, Santa Casa
Hospital Complex, Porto Alegre, Brazil;
Clinica da Mao ao Cotovelo, Porto Alegre, Rio
Grande, Brazil

RICHARD SMITH, PhD
Associate Professor, Department of
Orthopaedic Surgery and Biomedical
Engineering, University of Tennessee-
Campbell Clinic, Memphis, Tennessee,
USA

BRYAN D. SPRINGER, MD
Associate Professor, OrthoCarolina Hip
and Knee Center, Atrium Health
Musculoskeletal Institute, Charlotte, North
Carolina, USA

RAMESH C. SRINIVASAN, MD
Hand Center of San Antonio, Department of
Orthopaedic Surgery, UT San Antonio, San
Antonio, Texas, USA

THOMAS W. THROCKMORTON, MD
Professor, Department of Orthopaedic
Surgery and Biomedical Engineering,
University of Tennessee-Campbell Clinic,
Memphis, Tennessee, USA

LUKE TIDWELL, MS
Medical Student, Department of Orthopaedic
Surgery and Biomedical Engineering,

University of Tennessee-Campbell Clinic, Memphis, Tennessee, USA

JORDAN D. WALTERS, MD
Resident, Department of Orthopaedic Surgery and Biomedical Engineering, University of

Tennessee-Campbell Clinic, Memphis, Tennessee, USA

S. CLIFTON WILLIMON, MD
Children's Healthcare of Atlanta, Atlanta, Georgia, USA

CONTENTS

Knee and Hip Reconstruction
Patrick C. Toy and William M. Mihalko

> Using an age- and comorbidity-matched cohort, we compared patients who
> underwent unicompartmental knee arthroplasty in an ambulatory surgery cen-
> ter with those who underwent the procedure in a traditional hospital inpatient
> setting. Postoperatively, the ambulatory surgery center cohort had fewer major
> complications than the inpatient cohort. No ambulatory surgery center patients
> required acute hospital admission and none had major complications. Four
> major complications occurred in the inpatient cohort. There was no difference
> in complication rates. Our results suggest that outpatient unicompartmental
> knee arthroplasty in a freestanding ambulatory surgery center is a safe and
> reasonable alternative to the traditional inpatient hospital setting.

> Surgical techniques used to decrease the amount of blood lost during the
> procedure range from tourniquets to electrocautery and, more recently,
> the use of antifibrinolytics. Currently, tranexamic acid is the most commonly
> used antifibrinolytic in arthroplasty procedures. It was previously thought that
> intravenous tranexamic acid was more effective than topical tranexamic acid,
> but had an increased risk of thrombosis and cardiac events; however, this
> study showed that topical tranexamic acid is as effective in decreasing blood
> loss and the need for a blood transfusion after hybrid fixation total knee
> arthroplasty as with cemented total knee arthroplasty.

Trauma
John C. Weinlein and Michael J. Beebe

> Open reduction and internal fixation of displaced acetabular fractures has been
> the gold standard for treatment of these complex injuries. The subset of older
> patients with dome impaction, femoral head impaction, or a posterior wall
> component are considered for treatment with concomitant open reduction
> and internal fixation and total hip arthroplasty. Little has been written on the
> surgical techniques to perform concomitant open reduction and internal fixa-
> tion plus total hip arthroplasty safely. This article describes the important
> intrinsic factors for acetabular component stability, choice of surgical approach
> for management of these injuries, and surgical technique for anterior and pos-
> terior approaches.

Scapholunate ligament injuries are common and can lead to a predictable pattern of arthritis (scaphoid lunate advanced collapse wrist) if unrecognized or untreated. This article describes the relevant anatomy, biomechanics, and classification system, and provides an up-to-date literature-based review of treatment options, including acute repair and various reconstruction techniques. It also helps guide surgeons in making decisions regarding a systematic treatment algorithm for these injuries.

Shoulder and Elbow
Tyler J. Brolin

Proximal humeral bone loss in revision shoulder arthroplasty poses a significant obstacle to achieving stable and reliable fixation of the humeral stem. It is important to identify and classify this bone loss preoperatively, which can range from epiphyseal to substantial diaphyseal bone loss. There are several reconstructive options that can address the varying levels of bone loss, including cemented long-stem fixation, a composite construct using proximal humeral allograft or femoral allograft, proximal humeral endoprosthetic replacement, or total humeral replacement. All of these are viable reconstructive options that have demonstrated adequate to good outcomes.

Osteochondritis dissecans (OCD) of the capitellum is a relatively rare condition, occurring most frequently in adolescents who participate in repetitive overhead sports. The surgical treatment approach for this uncommon problem has varied from microfracture, loose body removal, abrasion chrondroplasty, lesion fixation, osteochondral allograft transplantation surgery, and osteochondral autologous transplantation surgery. The purpose of this study is to present the authors' preferred surgical technique for the treatment of unstable OCD lesions of the capitellum with osteochondral autologous transplantation surgery using autograft from the ipsilateral knee.

Foot and Ankle
Clayton C. Bettin and Benjamin J. Grear

Reconstruction of the flexible adult-acquired flatfoot deformity (AAFD) is controversial, and numerous procedures are frequently used in combination, including flexor digitorum longus transfer, medializing calcaneal osteotomy (MCO), heel cord lengthening/gastrocnemius recession, lateral column lengthening (LCL), Cotton osteotomy or first tarsometatarsal fusion, and spring ligament reconstruction. This article summarizes recent studies demonstrating that patients have significant improvements after operative treatment of flexible AAFD. It reviews current literature on clinical and radiographic outcomes of the MCO, LCL, and Cotton osteotomies. The authors describe how this information can be used in surgical decision making in order to tailor operative treatment to an individual patient's deformity.

Peroneal tendon pathology is becoming an increasingly recognized source of lateral-sided ankle pain. High clinical suspicion, along with judicious physical examination coupled with confirmatory advanced imaging modalities, are necessary to make an accurate diagnosis and aid in guiding treatment. Peroneal pathology encompasses several distinct conditions. Peroneal tendon tears and injuries to the peroneal retinaculum must be identified to guide treatment. Patients with peroneal pathology report high levels of satisfaction after surgical management with most returning to their preinjury level of function. An early and accurate diagnosis, along with treatment tailored to the individual, is necessary to obtain optimal outcomes.

RECONSTRUCTION

SERIES OF RELATED INTEREST

Clinics in Podiatric Medicine and Surgery
https://www.podiatric.theclinics.com/
Clinics in Sports Medicine
https://www.sportsmed.theclinics.com/
Foot and Ankle Clinics
https://www.foot.theclinics.com/
Hand Clinics
https://www.hand.theclinics.com/
Physical Medicine and Rehabilitation Clinics of North America
https://www.pmr.theclinics.com/

PREFACE

Reconstruction

Orthopedic "reconstruction" techniques, from total joint replacement to ligament reconstruction, encompass a variety of anatomic areas and musculoskeletal conditions. Innovative devices and techniques continue to improve outcomes and decrease complications and morbidity.

One area with major changes is total joint arthroplasty. The move from in-hospital to outpatient setting has transformed the experience of patients with total knee, hip, and shoulder procedures. Ford and colleagues compare unicompartmental knee arthroplasty procedures done in the ambulatory surgery center (ASC) to those done in the traditional in-hospital setting and found fewer complications in those done in the ASC, leading them to conclude that outpatient unicompartmental knee arthroplasty in a freestanding ASC is a safe and reasonable alternative to the traditional in-patient hospital setting. Techniques to reduce morbidity, including blood loss, also have aided in the move to outpatient arthroplasty. Chambers and colleagues investigate the use of topical tranexamic acid (TXA) in cemented and cementless total knee arthroplasty procedures and find that TXA is more effective in cementless arthroplasty.

Traumatic injuries, especially in elderly patients with poor bone quality, often require innovative repair or reconstruction techniques. Manson provides a detailed description of the technique for combining open reduction and internal fixation with total hip arthroplasty for treatment of displaced acetabular fractures in elderly patients. Rice and colleagues outline the indications for distal femoral replacement for treatment of fractures about the knee in elderly patients.

At the other end of the age spectrum, pediatric patients also may require reconstructive surgery. Treatment of slipped capital femoral epiphysis often results in residual deformity leading to femoroacetabular impingement (FAI) and eventually early-onset arthritis. Allen and Rosenfeld describe new surgical techniques for improving current symptoms of FAI and delaying or preventing hip arthritis. Increased sports participation has resulted in more frequent anterior cruciate ligament injuries in young patients, many of whom require ligament reconstruction. Perkins and Willimon outline indications for transphyseal and physeal-sparing techniques and discuss outcomes and complications of both.

The scaphoid is the most frequently injured carpal bone, and scaphoid fractures often require surgical fixation. Approximately 10% of scaphoid fractures progress to nonunions, and Borges and colleagues outline a decision-making process for determining appropriate treatment based primarily on the length of time the nonunion has been present. Scapholunate ligament injuries are common wrist injuries and can lead to arthritis if unrecognized or untreated. Mullikin and colleagues review treatment options and provide a systematic treatment algorithm for these injuries.

Proximal humeral bone loss can be a challenging problem in revision shoulder arthroplasty. Kahn and Chalmers emphasize the importance of identifying and classifying this bone loss and choosing the appropriate reconstructive procedure. They discuss several options depending on the level of bone loss. Osteochondritis dissecans (OCD) of the capitellum is a relatively uncommon condition that occurs primarily in adolescent overhead athletes. Morris and colleagues describe their surgical technique of osteochondral autologous transplantation for treatment of OCD lesions of the capitellum.

Although a number of reconstructive procedures of the foot and ankle are aimed at pediatric conditions, such as clubfoot, similar conditions in adults (flexible adult-acquired flatfoot deformity) also may require reconstruction. Conti and colleagues summarize current literature on treatment options and provide information for surgical

Orthop Clin N Am 51 (2020) xv–xvi
https://doi.org/10.1016/j.ocl.2019.10.001
0030-5898/20/© 2019 Published by Elsevier Inc.

decision making. Peroneal tendon pathology requires a high clinical suspicion, complete physical examination, and advanced imaging for diagnosis and treatment decisions, as discussed by Bahad and Kane. Most patients treated for peroneal tendon pathology are satisfied with their results and return to their preinjury function level.

For a variety of musculoskeletal conditions, orthopedists have moved beyond simply "repair" to "reconstruction." The authors in this issue have provided much useful information on choosing and implementing reconstruction techniques that produce the best outcomes for our patients.

Frederick M. Azar, MD
Professor, University of Tennessee–
Campbell Clinic
Department of Orthopaedic Surgery
1211 Union Avenue, Suite 510
Memphis, TN 38104, USA

E-mail address:
fazar@campbellclinic.com

Knee and Hip Reconstruction

Safety and Cost-Effectiveness of Outpatient Unicompartmental Knee Arthroplasty in the Ambulatory Surgery Center

A Matched Cohort Study

Marcus C. Ford, MD*, Jordan D. Walters, MD,
Ryan P. Mulligan, MD, Gregory D. Dabov, MD,
William M. Mihalko, MD, PhD, Anthony M. Mascioli, MD,
Thomas W. Throckmorton, MD

KEYWORDS

- Unicompartmental knee arthroplasty • Ambulatory surgery center • Outpatient procedure
- Outcomes • Complications

KEY POINTS

- There was no statistically significant difference in complication rates between the ambulatory surgery center and inpatient cohorts.
- The ambulatory surgery center allows the surgeon greater direct control of perioperative variables that can impact patient outcome.
- It has not been proven that the ambulatory surgery center is statistically safer than the hospital for unicompartmental knee arthroplasty.
- Outpatient unicompartmental knee arthroplasty in the ambulatory surgery center is a safe and reasonable alternative to unicompartmental knee arthroplasty in the traditional inpatient hospital setting.
- Patient selection is paramount when considering performing any procedure in the ambulatory surgery center.

Unicompartmental knee arthroplasty (UKA) has an established track record of providing pain relief and improving function in patients with unicompartmental osteoarthritis of the knee.[1–4] Reports demonstrate that shortened length of stay may decrease perioperative complications, heighten patient satisfaction, and decrease costs associated with arthroplasty procedures.[2,5–7] With a renewed emphasis on procedural safety, efficiency, and cost effectiveness, many surgeons

and patients are finding the ambulatory surgery center (ASC) a viable option for arthroplasty procedures.[2,5,8–11] Only a few reports in the literature describe UKA performed in an ASC with day-of-surgery discharge.[2,6,7,12–14]

The authors compared a matched cohort of outpatient UKAs performed in a freestanding ASC with those performed in the inpatient hospital setting to evaluate episode-of-care complications. Our hypothesis was that UKA

Department of Orthopaedic Surgery and Biomedical Engineering, University of Tennessee-Campbell Clinic, 1211 Union Avenue, Suite 510, Memphis, TN 38104, USA
* Corresponding author.
E-mail address: mford@campbellclinic.com

Orthop Clin N Am 51 (2020) 1–5
https://doi.org/10.1016/j.ocl.2019.08.001

is as safe as in the inpatient setting when done in a freestanding ASC with day-of-surgery discharge.

METHODS

After institutional review board approval, all data on UKA procedures performed by 2 board-certified orthopedic surgeons between 2009 and 2015 were reviewed retrospectively. None of the authors have financial or other conflicts that might have biased their work. A total of 150 medial, mobile-bearing UKAs were performed, 67 of which were done at a freestanding ASC. An age- and comorbidities-matched cohort included 48 patients who had UKA in the standard inpatient hospital setting. Ninety-day episode of care measures included complications, hospital (re)admissions, and reoperations. Statistical differences ($P<.05$) between the ASC and inpatient groups were determined by 2-tailed t-tests.

Perioperative Pathway

Patients with medial unicompartmental osteoarthritis of the knee in whom exhaustive nonoperative treatment failed to relieve symptoms were considered candidates for UKA. Preoperatively, all patients were evaluated with standing and valgus stress radiographs. Patients in whom valgus stress did not correct alignment to neutral and patients whose radiographs demonstrated arthritic changes in the lateral, posteromedial, or patellofemoral compartments were not considered candidates for UKA. Clinically, all patients were evaluated for anterior cruciate ligament integrity along with appropriate range of motion.

All patients were evaluated by a primary care physician and an anesthesiologist before surgery. Only patients with American Society of Anesthesiologists (ASA) scores of I, II, or III were considered UKA surgical candidates. All patients were thoroughly counseled about postoperative expectations. In preparation for surgery, all patients visited with physical therapy, and each was given a UKA information booklet. In addition, each patient's social and support systems were investigated.

Preoperatively, all patients were given a long-acting narcotic (typically extended release oxycodone), a nonsteroidal anti-inflammatory drug (typically celecoxib), a neurologic agent (typically gabapentin), dexamethasone, and oral acetaminophen unless contraindicated. All patients were given weight-based cefazolin immediately before surgery unless contraindicated.

Surgical Technique

Spinal anesthesia was used in most patients; general anesthesia was used for those in whom spinal anesthesia could not be obtained owing to anatomic limitations. Single-shot femoral nerve or adductor canal blocks were used in all patients. Unless contraindicated, intravenous tranexamic acid was used for hemostasis. In patients with a history of venous thromboembolism or stroke, topical tranexamic acid was used.

After tourniquet application, an anteromedial skin incision and a mini-medial parapatellar capsular incision were made with subluxation of the patella. The lateral and patellofemoral joints and the anterior cruciate ligament were inspected. Mobile-bearing medial UKA implants (Oxford Knee, Biomet, Warsaw, IN) were used in all patients.

After the final implants were cemented in place and before capsular closure, all periarticular tissues were locally injected with anesthetic. After injection, hemostasis was achieved, the capsule and soft tissues were closed, and a bulky dressing was placed. No drains were used.

Postoperative Protocol

Postoperatively, all patients in both cohorts were given short-acting narcotics (typically oxycodone–acetaminophen) and continued on NSAIDs and neurologic agents if not contraindicated. Short-acting intravenous narcotics and antiemetic agents were available before discharge. Patients deemed to be low risk for deep venous thrombosis were prescribed aspirin twice a day postoperatively for venous thromboembolism prophylaxis, whereas patients deemed to be at higher risk were placed on 14 days of low-molecular-weight heparin once daily followed by one additional month of twice daily aspirin.

In the ASC group, all patients were mobilized by a trained registered nurse as soon as medically possible. Clearance by both the surgeon and anesthesiologist were required before discharge on the day of surgery. All patients were discharged home with a rolling walker (or crutches) and home therapy instructions. In the event that a patient failed to meet accelerated postoperative discharge criteria, there was an available 23-hour observation room in the ASC.

In the hospital group, physical therapy was started on the afternoon of surgery and twice daily thereafter. Mechanical foot pumps were used in addition to the chemical venous thromboembolism prophylaxis protocol during the hospital stay. Clearance by physical therapy and the surgeon was required before discharge.

After discharge, all patients (ASC and hospital) had outpatient physical therapy three times per week. All patients were seen 10 to 14 days after surgery to assess their progress, and then again at 6 and 12 weeks postoperatively.

RESULTS

Forty-eight patients, matched based on age and associated comorbidities, were included in both the ASC and in-patient cohorts. The cohorts demonstrated no statistically significant differences in age (P = .55), sex (P = .40), body mass index (P = .29), or ASA physical status classification scores (P = .15) (Table 1).

No major complications were noted in patients in the ASC cohort. One minor complication occurred, a superficial stitch abscess. The overall complication rate for the ASC cohort was 2.1%. No patients in the ASC cohort required postoperative hospital admission, and no ASC cohort patients required reoperation within 90 days of surgery. All ASC cohort patients were discharged the same day of surgery without an overnight stay.

Four major complications were noted in the hospital cohort: 1 deep venous thrombosis, 1 pulmonary embolus, 1 acute postoperative infection, and 1 postoperative periprosthetic fracture. One minor complication was noted, a superficial skin allergic-type reaction. The overall complication rate for the hospital cohort was 10.4%. All 4 of the inpatient cohort patients with complications required hospital readmission (readmission rate 8.3%), whereas 2 required

reoperation (reoperation rate 4.2%). All patients with major complications had a preoperative ASA score of either II or III. The average length of stay for the hospital group was 2.9 days.

There was no statistically significant difference in complication rates between the ASC and inpatient matched cohorts (P = .2; Table 2).

DISCUSSION

As the population continues to age, the number of knee arthroplasty procedures continues to increase.[15] With a renewed emphasis on health care cost control, surgeons and patients alike seek to optimize treatment efficiency and cost effectiveness. Currently, focus is placed on decreasing length of stay and minimizing perioperative complications as major means to control costs.[2,16,17]

Arthroplasty procedures, including UKA, have traditionally been performed in the hospital inpatient setting. With advances in pain control and blood loss, traditional lengthy hospital stays became shorter inpatient hospital stays or even same-day or overnight discharges. More recently, many authors have reported the safety and success of outpatient total joint arthroplasty.[5–11] It is difficult, however, to define exactly the term outpatient, because it often includes patients who stay overnight and are discharged within 23 hours. Gondusky and colleagues[2] reported 160 patients who underwent UKA, 47 of whom were successfully discharged on the same day as surgery. No patients required overnight hospital admission on the day of surgery, and there were few 90-day episode-of-care complications. All patients demonstrated improved knee scores.

Our institution has been performing outpatient UKA in a freestanding ASC since 2009. Based on the subjective success of our UKA program in the ASC, we also have recently increased the number of total knee, total hip, and total shoulder arthroplasties performed in the ASC under strict inclusion criteria. To determine if our subjective impression was supported

Table 1			
Patient demographics and complications			
	ASC	Hospital	P value
Age (y)	58.8	59.4	.55
Sex			.40
Male	15 (31.3%)	20 (41.7%)	
Female	33 (68.7%)	28 (58.3%)	
Body mass index	34.3	32.9	.29
ASA	1.94	2.08	.15
Complications	1 (2.1%)	5 (10.4%)	.20
Minor	1 (2.1%)	1 (2.1%)	1.00
Major	0 (0.0%)	4 (8.3%)	.12
Reoperation	0 (0.0%)	2 (4.2%)	.49
Readmission	0 (0.0%)	4 (8.3%)	.12
Length of stay (d)	0	2.9	

Table 2	
Average total charges for UKA and TKA	
Location	Average Total Charges
ASC, Current study	$29,475.14 (UKA)
Nashville, TN	$37,859.09 (TKA)
Jackson, MS	$32,913.03 (TKA)
Fayetteville, AR	$26,129.04 (TKA)

Abbreviation: TKA, total knee arthroplasty.

by objective data, we analyzed the safety of UKA done in the ASC.

Based on an age- and comorbidity-matched cohort, we were able to compare patients who underwent UKA in the ASC with those who underwent the procedure in a traditional hospital inpatient setting. Both groups had similar preoperative ASA scores and body mass indexes (with the ASC group having a slightly higher body mass index). Postoperatively, the ASC cohort had fewer major complications than the inpatient cohort. None of the ASC patients required acute hospital admission and no ASC patients had major complications that required readmission or reoperation within the first 90 days after surgery. Four major complications occurred (8.3% major complication rate) in the inpatient cohort. There was no statistically significant difference in complication rates between the ASC and inpatient cohorts.

We believe that the ASC allows the surgeon greater direct control of perioperative variables that can impact patient outcome. We cannot say, however, that the ASC is statistically safer than the hospital for UKA. As more total joint procedures move to the ASC, larger randomized prospective studies may help to determine if the ASC is a safer place to perform UKA than the inpatient hospital setting. It also must be stressed that patient selection is paramount when considering performing any procedure in the ASC. In carefully selected patients, the ASC seems to be a safe alternative to the inpatient hospital setting.

There are some inherent weaknesses in this study. First, limited numbers do not allow for statistically significant safety comparisons between cohorts. We retrospectively investigated our data and evaluated only short-term outcomes up to 90 days postoperatively. We also did not evaluate functional scores or patient reported outcomes.

There is an inherent selection bias when determining those patients who are suitable for UKA in the ASC. Naturally, surgeons select those patients who are deemed physically and mentally capable of succeeding with an accelerated discharge plan. We chose to perform a matched cohort study to limit our selection bias as much as possible. Although government insurance programs currently do not restrict UKA procedures in the ASC, other arthroplasty procedures are restricted in older patients.

SUMMARY

Our results demonstrate that outpatient UKA in a freestanding ASC is a safe and reasonable alternative to UKA performed in the traditional inpatient hospital setting. Our institution's ASC total joint program initially began with UKA, and now has expanded to include total knee, hip and shoulder arthroplasties. Despite our favorable short-term results with UKA in the ASC, further investigation is required to definitively establish the long-term safety and cost-effectiveness of UKA performed in the ASC setting.

REFERENCES

1. Berger RA, Meneghini RM, Jacobs JJ, et al. Results of unicompartmental knee arthroplasty at a minimum of ten years follow up. J Bone Joint Surg Am 2005;87(5):999–1006.
2. Gondusky JS, Choi L, Khalaf N, et al. Day of surgery discharge after unicompartmental knee arthroplasty: an effective perioperative pathway. J Arthroplasty 2014;29(3):516–9.
3. Lyons MC, MacDonald SJ, Somerville LE, et al. Unicompartmental vs total knee arthroplasty database analysis: is there a winner? Clin Orthop Relat Res 2012;470(1):84–90.
4. Brown NM, Sheth NP, Davis K, et al. Total knee arthroplasty has higher postoperative morbidity than unicompartmental knee arthroplasty: a multicenter analysis. J Arthroplasty 2012;27(8 Suppl 1): 86–90.
5. Berger RA, Kusuma SK, Sanders SA, et al. The feasibility and perioperative complications of outpatient knee arthroplasty. Clin Orthop Relat Res 2009; 467(6):1443–9.
6. Bovonratwet P, Ondeck NT, Tyagi V, et al. Outpatient and inpatient unicompartmental knee arthroplasty procedures have similar short-term complication profiles. J Arthroplasty 2017;32(10):2935–40.
7. Cross MB, Berger R. Feasibility and safety of performing outpatient unicompartmental knee arthroplasty. Int Orthop 2014;38(2):443–7.
8. Lovald ST, Ong KL, Malkani AL, et al. Complications, mortality, and costs for outpatient and short-stay total knee arthroplasty patients in comparison to standard-stay patients. J Arthroplasty 2014;29(3):510–5.
9. Brolin TJ, Mulligan RP, Azar FM, et al. Neer Award 2016: outpatient total shoulder arthroplasty in an ambulatory surgery center is a safe alternative to inpatient total should arthroplasty in a hospital: a matched cohort study. J Shoulder Elbow Surg 2017;26:204–8.
10. Goyal N, Chen AF, Padgett SE, et al. Otto Aufranc Award: a multicenter, randomized study of outpatient versus in patient total hip arthroplasty. Clin Orthop Relat Res 2017;475:364–72.
11. Pollock M, Somerville L, Firth A, et al. Outpatient total hip arthroplasty, total knee arthroplasty, and

unicompartmental knee arthroplasty: a systematic review of the literature. JBJS Rev 2016;4(12) [pii: 01874474-201612000-00004].

12. Bradley B, Middleton S, Davis N, et al. Discharge on the day of surgery following unicompartmental knee arthroplasty within the United Kingdom NHS. Bone Joint J 2017;99-B(6):788–92.

13. Dervin GF, Madden SM, Crawford-Newton BA, et al. Outpatient unicompartmental knee arthroplasty with indwelling femoral nerve catheter. J Arthroplasty 2012;27(6):1159–65.

14. Kort NP, Bemelmans YFL, Schotanus MGM. Outpatient surgery for unicompartmental knee arthroplasty is effective and safe. Knee Surg Sports Traumatol Arthrosc 2017;25(9):2659–67.

15. Weinstein AM, Rome BN, Reichmann WM, et al. Estimating the burden of total knee replacement in the United States. J Bone Joint Surg Am 2013; 95(5):385–92.

16. Richter DL, Diduch DR. Cost comparison of outpatient versus inpatient unicompartmental knee arthroplasty. Orthop J Sports Med 2017;5(3). 2325967117694352.

17. Huang A, Ryu JJ, Dervin G. Cost savings of outpatient versus standard inpatient total knee arthroplasty. Can J Surg 2017;60(1):57–62.

Topical Tranexamic Acid Is Effective in Cementless Total Knee Arthroplasty

Stephen Chambers, MD, Luke Tidwell, MS,
Anita Kerkhof, MS, Richard Smith, PhD,
William M. Mihalko, MD, PhD*

KEYWORDS

- Total knee arthroplasty • Topical tranexamic acid • Blood loss • Transfusion
- Hybrid implant fixation

KEY POINTS

- Previous studies have shown that topical tranexamic acid is effective in decreasing the need for blood transfusion and decreasing blood loss in patients with cemented total knee arthroplasty.
- Few studies have investigated topical tranexamic acid use with hybrid fixation techniques.
- Although there remains some controversy surrounding the use of intravenous or topical tranexamic acid, recent studies have shown that they have similar effectiveness and complication rates.
- This study found that topical tranexamic acid is as effective in decreasing the rate of blood transfusions for total knee arthroplasty with hybrid fixation as with cemented fixation.
- Topical tranexamic acid decreases blood loss and has a protective role, even in hybrid fixation total knee arthroplasty where there is no barrier to blood loss in the bone implant interface.

Total knee arthroplasty (TKA) is an effective solution to restore function and relieve pain for patients with end-stage arthritis and is the one of the most common procedures performed in the United States, with approximately 700,000 done each year.[1] As this number continues to increase, so does the concern for reducing surgical complications and optimizing surgical techniques. With outpatient and 23-hour stays after primary TKA becoming more popular, the need to reduce blood loss is becoming more important.

The amount of blood lost during a TKA has a wide range of values.[2–6] This variability can be attributed to many different factors such as the use of a tourniquet, length of the procedure, type of implants, surgical technique, and specific patient factors (eg, genetics, preexisting hypercoagulable conditions, and even certain home medications). With increasing amounts of blood loss, patients have longer hospital stays, require blood transfusions, and have an overall increase in morbidity and mortality.[7,8] Transfusions have their own risks, including anaphylactic reactions and, in rare incidences, infections, as well as adding to the total cost of patient care.[9–12] Surgical techniques used to decrease the amount of blood lost during the procedure range from tourniquets to electrocautery and, more recently, the use of antifibrinolytics. Currently, tranexamic acid (TXA) is the most commonly used antifibrinolytic in arthroplasty procedures.[13,14] It was previously thought that intravenous TXA was more effective than topical TXA, but had an increased risk of thrombosis and cardiac events; however, several studies have shown that topical TXA is just as effective as

Department of Orthopaedic Surgery and Biomedical Engineering, University of Tennessee-Campbell Clinic, 1211 Union Avenue, Suite 510, Memphis, TN 38104, USA
* Corresponding author.
E-mail address: wmihalko@campbellclinic.com

Orthop Clin N Am 51 (2020) 7–11
https://doi.org/10.1016/j.ocl.2019.08.002
0030-5898/20/© 2019 Elsevier Inc. All rights reserved.

systemic TXA in decreasing blood loss, with no difference in thrombotic events.[2,15–19]

TKA fixation techniques also have an effect on the amount of blood lost during a procedure.[20–26] Although most surgeons use cemented fixation (CF) for primary TKA, there are a growing number of surgeons who use press-fit fixation on one (typically the femoral) component, termed hybrid fixation (HF), or both implants. Cementless fixation means that there is no barrier to keep the cancellous bone implant interface from losing blood after the procedure. Few studies have compared HF and CF in relation to blood loss[22,24,27]; these studies did not include the use of TXA. Our study focused on blood loss and subsequent transfusion requirements in patients with TKA with hybrid implant fixation, with and without topical TXA. We hypothesized that patients receiving TXA would have higher postoperative hematocrit levels and, therefore, require fewer transfusions.

METHODS

After institutional review board approval, this retrospective study was performed at a local Veterans Administration hospital from 2015 to 2017. Inclusion criteria were age 18 or over, primary total knee replacement with HF, and non-traumatic end-stage osteoarthritis. Patients were excluded if they had preexisting coagulopathy disorders (genetic, international normalized ratio of >1.2 or thrombocytopenia [150,000/mm^3], chronic anemia [defined as hemoglobin <10 g/dL preoperatively]), complications during surgery, and revision arthroplasty. Patients who required blood transfusion during the procedure also were excluded. Patients on preexisting anticoagulation medicine (such as aspirin and warfarin) were told to stop their medication at least 5 to 10 days before the surgery. To help control for variations in surgical technique, patients of only 1 surgeon were studied.

SURGICAL TECHNIQUE

In all patients, a tourniquet was inflated to 275 mm of pressure before skin incision. All surgeries used a standard medial parapatellar approach using the same implants. After component fixation and before fascial closure, 2 g of topical TXA in 100 mL of saline was applied and allowed to sit for 5 minutes. The tourniquet was then released, hemostasis was achieved, and a 10F Hemovac drain was placed. The drain was removed on postoperative day 1. The choice of TXA use was based on the timing of

implementation into the surgeon's practice. Postoperatively, all patients followed similar protocols for anticoagulation (enoxaparin) and fluid resuscitation. Blood transfusion was indicated for a postoperative hemoglobin level of less than 7 g/dL or symptoms such as orthostatic hypotension. Hospital records were used to determine the number of blood transfusions required, intraoperative blood loss, and postoperative drainage, and preoperative and postoperative day 2 hemoglobin levels. A Pearson χ^2 test was used for statistical analysis.

RESULTS

Chart review identified 139 patients with primary TKA who met inclusion criteria, 92 HF patients and 47 CF patients. Patients were then subclassified according to whether or not they received topical TXA (Table 1).

Transfusions

No transfusions were required in patients in the HF or CF group who received topical TXA (52 patients), compared with 6 (6.8%) in the 87 HF or CF patients without TXA (P = .053). When taking into account the type of fixation, none of 32 patients in the HF group with TXA required a transfusion, compared with 5 (8.3%) transfusions in the 60 HF patients without TXA (P = .093).

Blood Loss

Blood loss was calculated using the difference in preoperative and postoperative day 2 hemoglobin levels (Table 2). Topical TXA in both CF and HF patients had an overall protective effect on blood loss when compared with the non-TXA CF and HF combined group, with a mean preoperative minus postoperative hemoglobin of 2.5 g/dL for TXA group compared with a mean of 3.1 g/dL for non-TXA group at postoperative day 2 (P = .001). Without the use of TXA, both HF and CF groups showed a greater

Table 1
Topical TXA use in patients with hybrid and CF

Topical TXA	Hybrid[a]	Implant Type Cemented	Total
Yes	32 (62%)	20 (38%)	52 (100%)
No	60 (69%)	27 (31%)	87 (100%)
Total	92	47	139

[a] HF – press-fit femoral component and cemented tibial component.

Table 2
Results of topical TXA use in hybrid and CF

Topical TXA	Hybrid[a]	Cemented	Total
Number of patients requiring a transfusion			
Yes	0/32	0/20	0/52
No	5/60	1/27	6/86
Difference in preoperative and postoperative day 2 hemoglobin, g/dL (SD)			
Yes	2.41 (±0.77)	2.64 (±0.82)	2.5 (±0.79)
No	3.03 (±0.89)	3.44 (±0.95)	3.24 (±0.93)

[a] HF – press-fit femoral component and cemented tibial component.

difference in blood loss compared with TXA. In the patients in the HF without TXA group who required transfusion, the average postoperative day 2 difference in hemoglobin level was 3.45 g/dL, and in the 1 patient with CF without TXA who required a transfusion the difference was 4.3 g/dL.

There was also a significantly higher mean blood loss ($P = .03$) in the Hemovac group, with more blood loss in those not having TXA (199 mL) compared with those receiving TXA (73 mL).

DISCUSSION

Previous studies have shown that topical TXA is effective in reducing the need for blood transfusion and decreasing blood loss in patients with CF TKA.[1,15,16,18–20,28,29] There are, however, fewer studies that investigate topical TXA use with HF techniques.[21,24,27,30] Our results confirmed our hypothesis that topical TXA decreases blood loss and has a protective role even in HF TKA where there is no barrier to blood loss in the bone implant interface.

Given the increasing number of TKAs expected in the future, the use of topical TXA in TKA with HF can have a significant impact. Although there remains some controversy surrounding the use of intravenous or topical TXA, multiple recent studies have shown that they have similar effectiveness and complication rates.[16,18,30,31] Abdel and colleagues,[2] in a randomized controlled trial involving 620 patients, showed that the route of TXA administration was not a risk factor for a thrombolic event, and others have shown that topical TXA is safe for patients at high risk for VTE.[32–34] Some authors have suggested that topical TXA may be preferable to IV TXA because of ease of administration, cost effectiveness, and safety.[23,30]

The primary limitation of this study is the small sample size. A larger population would show quantitatively how effective topical TXA is with HF compared with CF. Another limitation is the difference in surgical technique for CF and HF, which may affect the amount of blood loss. Some investigators have suggested that cemented femoral components may have a tamponade effect or a cauterization effect from the exothermic reaction of the cement polymerization.[35–37] However, this finding was not consistent with our study in which the cemented group had overall more blood loss, which we cannot account for given the same techniques used for both groups. We also cannot comment on the different routes of TXA application that are being used now such as oral administration, which is becoming more popular.

SUMMARY

This study demonstrated that topical TXA more effectively decreases blood loss and the need for a blood transfusion after HF TKA compared with CF TKA. We believe this is important to report because of the increasing number of surgeons using press-fit implants for TKA.

REFERENCES

1. Kurtz SM, Ong KL, Lau E, et al. Impact of the economic downturn on total joint replacement demand in the United States: updated projections to 2021. J Bone Joint Surg Am 2014;96: 624–30.
2. Abdel MP, Chalmers BP, Tauton MJ, et al. Intravenous versus topical tranexamic acid in total knee arthroplasty: both effective in a randomized clinical trial of 640 patients. J Bone Joint Surg Am 2019; 100:1023–9.
3. Good L, Peterson E, Lisander B. Tranexamic acid decreases external blood loss but not hidden blood loss in total knee replacement. Br J Anaesth 2003;90(5):596–9.
4. Prasad N, Padmanabhan V, Mullaji A. Blood loss in total knee arthroplasty: an analysis of risk factors. Int Orthop 2007;31:39–44.
5. Sehat KR, Evans RL, Newman JH. Hidden blood loss following hip and knee arthroplasty. Correct management of blood loss should take hidden loss into account. J Bone Joint Surg Br 2004;86(4): 561–5.
6. Wong J, Abrishami A, El Beheiry H, et al. Topical application of tranexamic acid reduces postoperative blood loss in total knee arthroplasty: a

randomized, controlled trial. J Bone Joint Surg Am 2010;92(15):2503–13.

7. Bernard AC, Davenport DL, Chang PK, et al. Intra-operative transfusion of 1 U to 2 U packed red blood cells is associated with increased 30-day mortality, surgical-site infection, pneumonia, and sepsis in general surgery patients. J Am Coll Surg 2009;208(5):931–7 [discussion: 938–9].

8. Browne JA, Adib F, Brown TE, et al. Transfusion rates are increasing following total hip arthroplasty: risk factors and outcomes. J Arthroplasty 2013; 28(Suppl):34–7.

9. Dwyre DM, Fernando LP, Holland PV. Hepatitis B, hepatitis C and HIV transfusion-transmitted infections in the 21st century. Vox Sang 2011;100(1): 92–8.

10. Fernandez MC, Gottlieb M, Menitove JE. Blood transfusion and postoperative infection in orthopedic patients. Transfusion 1992;32(4):318–22.

11. Kato H, Nakayama T, Uruma M, et al. A retrospective observational study to assess adverse transfusion reactions of patients with and without prior transfusion history. Vox Sang 2015;108(3):243–50.

12. Nichols CI, Vose JG. Comparative risk of transfusion and incremental total hospitalization cost for primary unilateral, bilateral, and revision total knee arthroplasty procedures. J Arthroplasty 2016; 31(3):583–9.e1.

13. Benoni G, Fredin H. Fibrinolytic inhibition with tranexamic acid reduces blood loss and blood transfusion after knee arthroplasty: a prospective, randomised, double-blind study of 86 patients. J Bone Joint Surg Br 1996;78(3):434–40.

14. Marra F, Rosso F, Bruzzone M, et al. Use of tranexamic acid in total knee arthroplasty. Joints 2016;4: 202–13.

15. Liu Y, Meng F, Yang G, et al. Comparison of intra-articular versus intravenous application of tranexamic acid in total knee arthroplasty: a meta-analysis of randomized controlled trials. Arch Med Sci 2017;13:533–40.

16. Meena S, Benazzo F, Dwivdei S, et al. Topical versus intravenous tranexamic acid in total knee arthroplasty. J Orthop Surg (Hong Kong) 2017; 25(1). 2309499016684300.

17. Montroy J, Hutton B, Moodley P, et al. The efficacy and safety of topical tranexamic acid: a systematic review and meta-analysis. Transfus Med Rev 2018 [pii:S0887-7963(17)30151-7]. [Epub ahead of print].

18. Patel JN, Spanyer JM, Smith LS, et al. Comparison of intravenous versus topical tranexamic acid in total knee arthroplasty: a prospective randomized study. J Arthroplasty 2014;29:1528–31.

19. Tzatzairis TK, Drosos GI, Kotsios SE, et al. Intravenous vs topical tranexamic acid in total knee arthroplasty without tourniquet application: a randomized controlled study. J Arthroplasty 2016;31:2465–70.

20. Baker PN, Khaw FM, Kirk LM, et al. A randomised controlled trial of cemented versus cementless press-fit condylar total knee replacement: 15-year survival analysis. J Bone Joint Surg Br 2007;89:1608–14.

21. Christodoulou AG, Ploumis AL, Terzidis IP, et al. The role of timing of tourniquet release and cementing on perioperative blood loss in total knee replacement. Knee 2004;11:313–7.

22. Demey G, Servien E, Pinaroli A, et al. The influence of femoral cementing on perioperative blood loss in total knee arthroplasty: a prospective randomized study. J Bone Joint Surg Am 2010;92:536–41.

23. Ishii Y, Matsuda Y. Perioperative blood loss in cementless or hybrid total knee arthroplasty without patellar resurfacing: a prospective, randomized study. J Arthroplasty 2005;20:972–6.

24. Kim YH, Park JW, Lim HM, et al. Cementless and cemented total knee arthroplasty in patients younger than fifty-five years. Which is better? Int Orthop 2014;38:297–303.

25. Mylod AG Jr, France MP, Muser DE, et al. Perioperative blood loss associated with total knee arthroplasty. A comparison of procedures performed with and without cementing. J Bone Joint Surg Am 1990;72(7):1010–2.

26. Porteus AJ, Bartlett RJ. Post-operative drainage after cemented, hybrid and uncemented total knee replacement. Knee 2003;10:371–4.

27. Dorweiler MA, Boin MA, Froehle AW, et al. Improved early postoperative range of motion in total knee arthroplasty using tranexamic acid: a retrospective analysis. J Knee Surg 2019;32(2): 160–4.

28. Subramanyam KN, Khanchandani P, Tulajaprasad PV, et al. Efficacy and safety of intra-articular versus intravenous tranexamic acid in reducing perioperative blood loss in total knee arthroplasty: a prospective randomized double-blind equivalence trial. Bone Joint J 2018;100-B:152–60.

29. Ishii Y, Noguchi H, Sato J, et al. Effect of a single injection of tranexamic acid on blood loss after primary hybrid TKA. Knee 2015;22:197–200.

30. George J, Eachempati KK, Subramanyam KN, et al. The comparative efficacy and safety of topical and intravenous tranexamic acid for reducing perioperative blood loss in total knee arthroplasty: a randomized controlled non-inferiority trial. Knee 2018;25:185–91.

31. Mi B, Liu G, Lv H, et al. Is combined use of intravenous and intraarticular tranexamic acid superior to intravenous or intraarticular tranexamic acid alone in total knee arthroplasty? A meta-analysis of randomized controlled trials. J Orthop Surg Res 2017;12:61.

32. Delanois RE, Gwam C, Mistry JB, et al. Intraarticular administration of tranexamic acid is safe and effective in total knee arthroplasty patients at high-risk

for thromboembolism. Surg Technol Int 2016;30:
279–83.

33. Sabbag OD, Abdel MP, Amundson AW, et al. Tranexamic acid was safe in arthroplasty patients with a history of venous thromboembolism: a matched outcome study. J Arthroplasty 2017;32:S246–50.

34. Spanyer J, Patel J, Emberson E, et al. Topical tranexamic acid in total knee arthroplasty patients with increased thromboembolic risk. J Knee Surg 2017;30:474–8.

35. Charnley J. The reaction of bone to self-curing acrylic cement. A long-term histological study in man. J Bone Joint Surg Br 1970;52:340–53.

36. Jefferiss CD, Lee AJ, Ling RS. Thermal aspects of self-curing polymethyl-methacrylate. J Bone Joint Surg Br 1975;57:511–8.

37. Tronzo RG, Kallos T, Wyche MQ. Elevation of intramedullary pressure when methylmethacrylate is inserted in total hip arthroplasty. J Bone Joint Surg Am 1974;56:714–8.

Trauma

Open Reduction and Internal Fixation Plus Total Hip Arthroplasty for the Acute Treatment of Older Patients with Acetabular Fracture
Surgical Techniques

Theodore T. Manson, MD, MS

KEYWORDS

- Acetabular fracture • Open reduction and internal fixation • Total hip arthroplasty • Geriatric
- Levine (direct anterior) hip approach • Kocher-Langenbeck approach

---

KEY POINTS

- Open reduction and internal fixation plus concomitant total hip arthroplasty is an excellent treatment for older patients with selected acetabular fractures.
- The main goal of surgery is to restore the relationship between the ischium and anterior inferior iliac spine to allow for acetabular component stability.
- In selected posterior wall fractures, total hip arthroplasty alone can be used without concomitant open reduction and internal fixation.
- Depending on the location of the fracture and associated comminution, either a direct anterior (Levine) approach to the acetabulum or Kocher-Langenbeck approach to the acetabulum can be used.

INTRODUCTION

Open reduction and internal fixation (ORIF) of displaced acetabular fractures has been the gold standard for treatment of these complex injuries.[1,2] However, older patients with acetabular dome impaction,[3] femoral head impaction,[4,5] or a posterior wall component to their injury[6] have historically done poorly with standard ORIF techniques. This subset of older patients with dome impaction, femoral head impaction or a posterior wall component are who we consider for treatment with concomitant ORIF and total hip arthroplasty (THA) through the same incision.

To date, several retrospective series have detailed the results of combined ORIF + THA.[7–19] We have also recently completed a randomized controlled trial of ORIF versus ORIF + THA for patients older than 60 with displaced acetabular fractures with dome impaction or femoral head impaction or posterior wall fracture.[20] However little has been written on the surgical techniques to perform concomitant ORIF + THA safely.

The author presents his approach here, which was developed at the R. Adams Cowley Shock Trauma Center in Baltimore, Maryland, and then tested in a randomized controlled trial

---

Disclosure Statement: This research was funded by a generous grant from the Orthopaedic Research and Education Foundation.
Department of Orthopaedic Surgery, R Adams Cowley Shock Trauma Center, 8322 Bellona Avenue, Suite 100, Baltimore, MD 21204, USA
E-mail address: tmanson@towsonortho.com

Orthop Clin N Am 51 (2020) 13–26
https://doi.org/10.1016/j.ocl.2019.08.006
0030-5898/20/

comparing ORIF with ORIF plus concomitant THA in older patients with acetabular fracture.[20] The discussion is broken down into a description of the important intrinsic factors for acetabular component stability, choice of surgical approach for management of these injuries, and finally the details of surgical technique for anterior and posterior approaches.

WHAT BONY LANDMARKS ARE IMPORTANT FOR ACETABULAR COMPONENT STABILITY?

The goal of combined ORIF + THA is not to achieve a meticulous anatomic joint reduction, but to give a supportive bed for the acetabular component. A fully intact acetabulum is not always necessary to achieve stability of the acetabular component. The 2 most important bony landmarks for acetabular component stability are the subchondral bone attached to the anterior inferior iliac spine (AIIS) and the subchondral bone attached to the ischium (Fig. 1). The bone attached to the posterior wall of the acetabulum and the bone of the anterior wall of the acetabulum just lateral to the iliopectineal eminence are not as critical for stability of the acetabular component (Fig. 1).

Borrowing from principles of revision THA, the surgical goal is to wedge a multihole acetabular component between 2 points, the subchondral bone attached to the ischium and the subchondral bone attached to the AIIS (see Fig. 1). The relationship between the AIIS and ischium must be stable for this strategy to be successful. When using a Kocher-Langenbeck

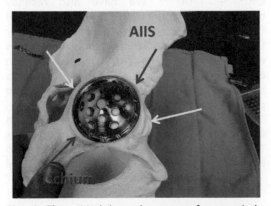

Fig. 1. The critical bony buttresses for acetabular component stability are the subchondral bone attached to the AIIS and the subchondral bone attached to the ischium (both represented with *red arrows*). The posterior wall and the anterior wall adjacent to the iliopectineal eminence are not as critical for component stability (*yellow arrows*). (*Courtesy of* T. Manson, MD, Baltimore, MD.)

Approach, this is usually achieved by one or two 3.5-mm reconstruction plates that span the posterior column of the acetabulum. When using the Levine (anterior) approach, this is usually accomplished using long 3.5-mm reconstruction plate along the pelvic brim and then long 3.5-mm or 7.3-mm screws that traverse from the anterior to the posterior column.

Careful evaluation of the preoperative computed tomography scan allows the surgeon to determine whether concomitant ORIF plus THA is necessary or whether THA alone can be used to manage the injury.

IS OPEN REDUCTION AND INTERNAL FIXATION ALWAYS NECESSARY BEFORE TOTAL HIP ARTHROPLASTY?

In the majority of cases, the relationship between the AIIS and the ischium will be disrupted by the acetabular fracture. Transverse fractures, anterior column fractures, associated both column injuries, anterior column-posterior hemitransverse, T-type, and posterior column fractures all fall into this category. In these cases, it is preferable to stabilize this relationship using acetabular fixation before reaming and placing the acetabular component.

The one relatively common exception is an isolated posterior wall fracture (Fig. 2). Many posterior wall fractures, even comminuted ones, leave the relationship between the AIIS and the ischium intact. Even in the face of marked posterior wall marginal impaction and comminution, if the subchondral bone attached to the ischium is intact ORIF may not be necessary before THA (Figs. 3–5).

Careful scrutiny of the preoperative computed tomography scan can assess whether

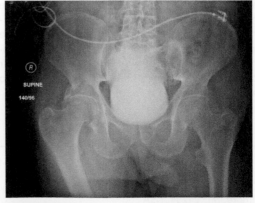

Fig. 2. An elderly patient with a posterior wall fracture dislocation sustained in a motor vehicle collision. (*Courtesy of* T. Manson, MD, Baltimore, MD.)

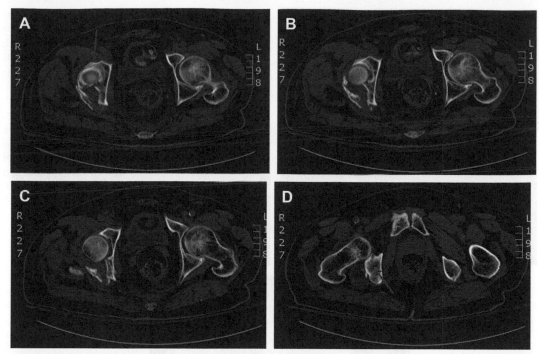

Fig. 3. The CT scan of the patient shown in **Fig. 2**. (*A*) Axial computed tomography image showing the subchondral bone attached to the AIIS is intact (*red arrow*). (*B, C*) Axial images from further distal shows a markedly comminuted posterior wall fracture. (*D*) Imaging of the lower acetabulum and ischium however shows that the subchondral bone attached to the inferior acetabulum and ischium is intact (*red arrow*). The surgical goal is to wedge the acetabular component between the AIIS and the ischium. (*Courtesy of* T. Manson, MD, Baltimore, MD.)

the ischium is supportive (see **Fig. 3**). In these cases, placement of an acetabular component, although not specifically addressing the posterior wall fracture, can be accomplished with bone grafting of the posterior wall defect using femoral head autograft (see **Figs. 4** and **5**).

In some posterior wall acetabular fractures, the piriformis, gemelli, and obturator internus may be torn and disrupted as a result of the injury. However, the obturator externus attachment to the posterior trochanter and the quadratus femoris attachment to the posterior greater trochanter are almost always left intact with these types of injuries. These are important stabilizers of a hip replacement postoperatively. Intuitively then, a surgeon could perform the hip replacement alone and leave these posterior structures intact through a direct anterior or Hardinge approach to the hip and exploit the natural increased stability of these approaches.[7,21]

SURGICAL TECHNIQUE FOR TOTAL HIP ARTHROPLASTY ALONE THROUGH AN ANTERIOR APPROACH FOR POSTERIOR WALL FRACTURES

The author typically uses the direct anterior approach to the hip when using THA alone for treatment of a posterior wall acetabular fracture. One of the benefits of this strategy is supine positioning of the patient. Supine positioning improves anesthesia staff access to the patient. Preparation and draping of both legs also allows for direct leg length comparison.

For acetabular preparation, we usually medialize to the floor of the cotyloid fossa first using a reamer 5 mm below our templated acetabular component size. We then ream the acetabulum for a 1 mm press fit for a hemispherical component. A trial acetabular component is used to confirm that we can wedge our implant between the subchondral bone attached to the AIIS and the subchondral bone attached to the ischium. Bone defects are grafted with bone from the native femoral head.

Our standard component used for this procedure is a multihole revision acetabular component. The component is impacted and the position checked using the transverse acetabular ligament and fluoroscopy as a guide. We typically uses 3 to 5 screws for acetabular component stabilization and these screws are placed superior and inferior to the equator of the acetabular component to prevent failure of the acetabular component in abduction (see **Figs. 4** and **5**).

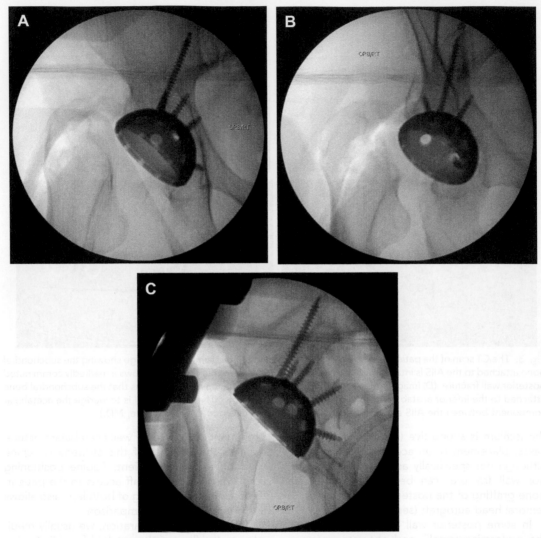

Fig. 4. (A) An anterior posterior fluoroscopic view taken during a direct anterior approach for the same patient shows a multihole acetabular component stabilized between the AIIS and ischium. Long screws are placed superior and inferior to the equator of the acetabular component. (B) An obturator oblique view taken during the direct anterior hip replacement shows multiple screws that are within the acetabular columns. A long screw traverses superiorly adjacent to the sciatic buttress. The posterior wall fracture has been impaction grafted but no direct reduction or fixation has been performed. (C) An iliac oblique view taken during the direct anterior hip replacement shows the long superior screw as well as multiple inferior screws that are headed posteriorly within the confines of the posterior column and ischium. (Courtesy of T. Manson, MD, Baltimore, MD.)

The femoral stem is then implanted using standard direct anterior technique. With the final components in place, leg length assessment is completed by comparing the lengths of the heels and medial malleoli. Both feet need to be centered underneath the pubic symphysis in order for this to be accurate (Fig. 6). Because the leg is draped free, the standard tests of hip impingement in deep flexion and internal rotation as well as external rotation and extension can also be performed. Fluoroscopic assessment of leg length equalization can also be used.[22]

Postoperative Care

The reconstruction gained by these techniques is very stable. To date, we have held patients touchdown or 50% weight bearing for 6 weeks postoperatively. Realistically, however, consideration could be given to full weight bearing immediately postoperatively based on surgeon discretion. We do not use any specific hip

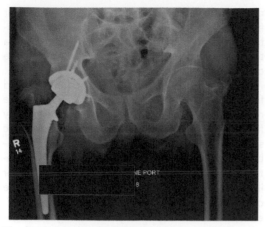

Fig. 5. The postoperative view shows a standard uncemented stem and uncemented multi hole acetabular component. (*Courtesy of* T. Manson, MD, Baltimore, MD.)

precautions, but do limit straight leg raise strengthening postoperatively to avoid iliopsoas tendon irritation.

IN CASES WHERE OPEN REDUCTION AND INTERNAL FIXATION IS REQUIRED

In fractures more complex than a posterior wall where the bony relationship between the AIIS and ischium is disrupted, ORIF is required before acetabular component placement. If the majority of the fracture displacement and comminution is anterior then we typically use an anteriorly based approach for combined ORIF + THA. If the majority of the fracture displacement and comminution is posterior then we typically use a Kocher-Langenbeck approach for ORIF + THA. We outline both approaches for ORIF + THA elsewhere in this article.

The focus is on speed of reduction and implant placement to minimize the risk of infection. Long operative times are associated with a dramatic increase in infection risk in hip arthroplasty.[23,24] The surgical goal is rapid reduction with bone stock stabilization rather than painstaking anatomic reduction.

OPEN REDUCTION AND INTERNAL FIXATION PLUS TOTAL HIP ARTHROPLASTY THROUGH AN ANTERIOR (LEVINE) APPROACH TO THE ACETABULUM

Levine in the 1940s[25] described the anterior intrapelvic approach as an extension of the Smith-Peterson interval for the management of

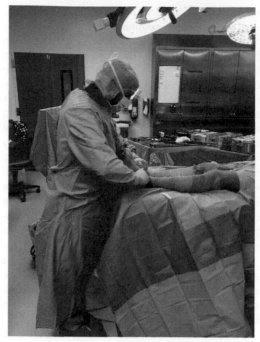

Fig. 6. Direct comparison of leg lengths by comparing both heels and medial malleoli together. Having an assistant mark the position of the pubic symphysis allows the surgeon to center the feet in the midline (critical for this technique to be accurate). (*Courtesy of* T. Manson, MD, Baltimore, MD.)

central acetabular fractures with protrusion. Beaulé and associates[7] revisited this approach in the early 2000s for concomitant ORIF plus THA. This approach gives direct access to the AIIS, anterior acetabulum and any associated comminution. However, patients must be carefully chosen for this approach based on the fracture patterns.

Indications
The best patients for an anterior approach for ORIF plus THA have comminution or fracture lines that disrupt the subchondral bone attached to the AIIS. The AIIS comminution can be difficult to address from a posterior approach to the hip. Many acetabular fractures in older patients involve protrusio with disruption of the quadrilateral surface and AIIS. Often, the posterior column of the acetabulum (if involved in the fracture) does not show a large degree of displacement. These are patients for whom an anterior approach may be ideal.

Surgical Technique
The patient is positioned supine for this procedure. A Hanna table may be used or a regular flat top radiolucent table such as a Jackson or OSI

table (Mizuho, Union City, CA) may be used. At our center, for routine direct anterior hip replacement, we use a regular operating room bed. However, most regular operating room beds will not allow visualization of an iliac oblique radiographs owing to interference with fluoroscopic imaging by the bed side rail. For this reason, we use a flat top table with the torso and buttocks raised up on blankets during the combined ORIF + THA procedure (Fig. 7). Early in our experience, we placed the patient's torso on folded blankets to allow for hyperextension of the hip during femoral preparation (see Fig. 7). However, the femoral exposure in these cases is much easier than for osteoarthritic patients so we now place the patient's torso directly on the radiolucent table.

Both legs are draped into the field. The hip as well as the area above the pubic symphysis are draped into the operative fields so that if necessary a Stoppa anterior intrapelvic approach can be made without re prep and drape (Fig. 8).

A standard direct anterior hip incision 2 to 3 cm lateral to the anterior superior iliac spine is extended proximally curving posteriorly over the iliac crest (see Fig. 8). We usually perform the direct anterior approach to the hip first. The tensor fascia lata sheath is split in its midline so as to protect the lateral femoral cutaneous nerve (Fig. 9A). The branches of the ascending branch of the lateral femoral circumflex artery are located and coagulated and an anterior capsulotomy is made exposing the femoral neck and head. At this point in time, the femoral neck and head may be left in place or they can be resected to facilitate reduction of the acetabular fracture. To equalize leg lengths postoperatively, the neck resection is based on a templated marker ball radiographs of the contralateral intact hip.

With the hip exposed, the dissection is carried further up to the anterior superior iliac spine. We release the inguinal ligament subperiosteally from its insertion on the anterior superior iliac spine and tag the ligament insertion with Ethibond suture for later repair (Fig. 9B). Alternatively, an osteotomy of the anterior superior iliac spine can be made for bony repair at the conclusion the procedure. Early in our experience, we used osteotomy of the inguinal ligament and Sartorius insertion; however, we have moved to subperiosteal release with later direct repair using nonabsorbable suture through drill holes at the conclusion of the procedure.

The iliacus muscle is elevated subperiosteally from the internal surface of the iliac fossa. With the hip flexed to release tension on the neurovascular structures, retractors are placed over the pelvic brim into the true pelvis (Fig. 9C). The rectus femoris tendon is retracted medially and is not usually released (Fig. 9D).

Further visualization of the low anterior column and wall could be accomplished by release of the direct head of the rectus femoris tendon from the AIIS (Fig. 9E). We have found this to be rarely necessary but it certainly improves exposure.

The goal of pelvic stabilization is not anatomic reduction, but to stabilize the relationship between the AIIS and ischium. Commonly, a long

A

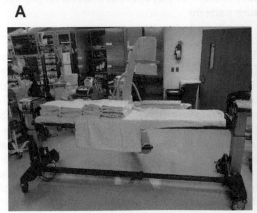

B

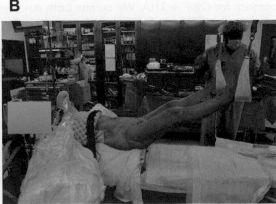

Fig. 7. (A) A standard flattop radiolucent table can be used for either anterior or posteriorly based approaches to the hip. Folded blankets placed underneath the patient's torso can facilitate hyperextension of the hip if using an anterior approach. (B) Patient preparation for concomitant ORIF plus THA through an anteriorly based approach. The patient's torso has been raised up off the operative table using folded blankets. This allows hyperextension of the hip; however, the author's current practice is to place the patient directly on a flat top radiolucent table and to prepare the femur without femoral hyperextension during the surgery. (*Courtesy of* T. Manson, MD, Baltimore, MD.)

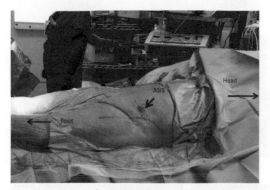

Fig. 8. Draping for concomitant ORIF plus THA through an anterior approach. The patient's head is to the right of the image and the foot is to the left of the image. An incision 3 fingerbreadths lateral to the anterior superior iliac spine curves proximally along the course of the iliac crest. (*Courtesy of* T. Manson, MD, Baltimore, MD.)

3.5-mm reconstruction plate is placed along the pelvic brim. To lock in the quadrilateral surface component of the fracture, long screws parallel to the quadrilateral surface traversing directly

medial to the fossa are very powerful for fixation of these fractures (**Fig. 10**).

Posterior column injuries can be reduced well through this approach as long as they are not significantly displaced. The posterior column component of the fracture can be stabilized with long 3.5- or 7.3-mm screws traversing from the iliac fossa into the posterior column (see **Fig. 10**). If there is significant quadrilateral surface comminution, the surgeon may use a separate Stoppa (anterior intrapelvic) approach to the acetabulum to stabilize this. This approach allows direct stabilization of the comminution with plates and screws applied directly medial to the quadrilateral surface (**Fig. 11**) In practice this is rarely necessary, but certainly feasible.

Acetabular Preparation

The acetabulum is reamed starting with a reamer about 5 mm smaller than the templated acetabular component size to the base of the cotyloid fossa. In general, we ream 1 mm under the acetabular component size chosen for a 1-mm press-fit.

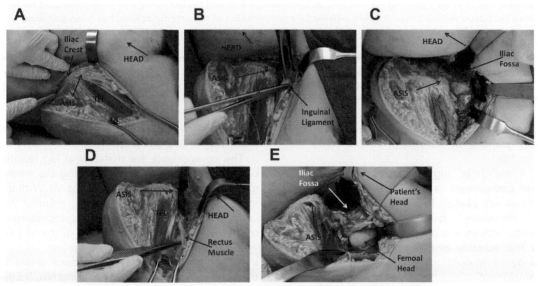

Fig. 9. (*A*) Cadaver dissection of a right-sided hip. The cadaver's head is to the left of the image. A standard incision is made in the midportion of the tensor fascia lata sheath and continues up to an incision over the iliac crest in between the external oblique fascia and the fascia lata. (*B*) Taking down the inguinal ligament from the anterior superior iliac spine (ASIS) connects the intrapelvic dissection and the dissection for the anterior hip replacement. The ligament is released in a subperiosteal fashion and tagged using a nonabsorbable suture. At the conclusion of the procedure, the inguinal ligament is usually repaired back down to the anterior superior iliac spine using Ethibond sutures through drill holes. (*C*) Exposure of the iliac fossa and pelvic brim without taking down the origin of the rectus femoris tendon. A spiked retractor can also be placed lateral to the iliopectineal eminence, as is typically performed in the approach for a Ganz acetabular osteotomy. (*D*) The direct head of the rectus muscle (end of the pickups) can be left attached to the AIIS. The rectus muscle is retracted medially and the reflected head of the rectus femoris is released as a surgeon would typically accomplish for a standard direct anterior hip replacement. (*E*) Release of the direct head of the rectus femoris insertion produces wide exposure of the hip and anterior acetabulum. This is rarely necessary in practice. TFL, tensor fascia latae. (*Courtesy of* T. Manson, MD, Baltimore, MD.)

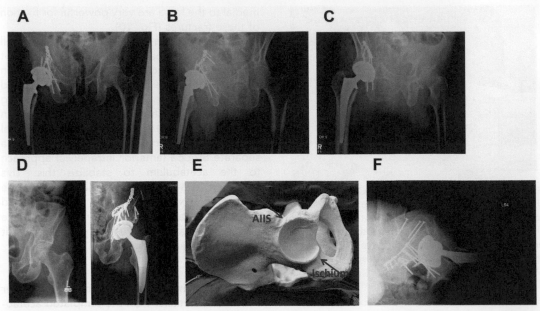

Fig. 10. (*A*) Postoperative anteroposterior pelvis radiograph shows fixation of a patient with an anterior column posterior hemitransverse fracture with long screws parallel to the quadrilateral surface stabilizing the relationship between the anterior and posterior columns of the acetabulum. (*B*) Postoperative iliac oblique view of the same patient shows the long screws parallel to the quadrilateral plate and medial to the acetabular component stabilizing the columns of the acetabulum. (*C*) Postoperative obturator oblique view of the same patient again shows the plate and long screws stabilizing the relationship between the AIIS and the ischium. (*D*) Another case used for illustrative purposes. An acetabular fracture with marked comminution of the anterior column has been stabilized with plates placed along the internal surface of the acetabulum stabilizing the relationship between the AIIS and the ischium. Bony osteotomies in this case were used to take down the inguinal ligament and rectus insertion for increased exposure. (*E*) The relationship between the AIIS and the ischium must be stable so that these 2 anatomic landmarks do not distract with impaction of the acetabular component. (*F*) A cross-table lateral view of the same patient in *D* demonstrates how long screws traversing in between the pelvic brim and the ischium stabilize the relationship between the AIIS and ischium as detailed in *E*. (*Courtesy of* T. Manson, MD, Baltimore, MD.)

Large bony defects are treated with impaction grafting of autograft femoral head (see **Fig. 15**).

A multihole, highly porous coated acetabular component is usually used and 4 to 5 screws are placed into the ilium, ischium, and if necessary quadrilateral surface and pubis. Screws are placed superior and inferior to the equator of the acetabular component to avoid abduction failure of the acetabular component.

Femoral Preparation

After fixation of the acetabulum, the femur is prepared by releasing the ischiofemoral ligament from the saddle area where the femoral neck joints the greater trochanter. Usually, the piriformis and external rotators can be left attached to the posterior aspect of the femur. In general, femoral elevation is more straightforward than in a direct anterior approach for osteoarthritis owing to the lack of capsular contracture, stiffness, and osteophytes. We do

not typically hyperextend the hip for femoral broaching or implant placement.

The components are trialed and leg lengths can be directly compared by placing the medial malleoli and heels together (see **Fig. 6**). With the final components in place, the anterior hip capsule is closed to the tendinous undersurface of the gluteus medius in the area of the saddle.

We typically repair the insertion of the inguinal ligament and sartorius back down to the anterior superior iliac spine using No. 5 Ethibond sutures and bony drill holes.

If the anterior superior iliac spine was taken off as an osteotomy, this is usually repaired using 3.5-mm screws.

The external oblique fascia is closed to the fascia lata over the iliac crest with a drain in the iliac fossa. The tensor fascia lata sheath is closed over a drain as well.

Postoperative Care

Patients are kept toe-touch weight bearing for 3 months postoperatively and then advanced

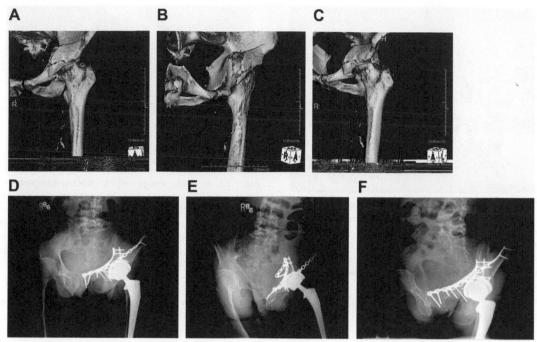

Fig. 11. (*A–C*) Anteroposterior, iliac, and obturator views taken from a 3-dimensional reconstruction of an older patient with an acetabular fracture show comminution of the AIIS and the subchondral bone in the acetabulum attached to it. (*D–F*) Anteroposterior, iliac, and obturator views show reconstruction of the AIIS and quadrilateral plate. In this case, an Anterior Intrapelvic Approach (AIP) or Stoppa approach was used for supplemental fixation. In the author's experience, this maneuver is rarely necessary, and most patients can be managed without a separate anterior intrapelvic approach. (*Courtesy of* T. Manson, MD, Baltimore, MD.)

slowly to weight bearing as tolerated with gradual relinquishment of assistant devices. Earlier weight bearing can probably be used, depending on the displacement and overall comminution present in the posterior column. However, in our center we have not moved to the use of earlier weight bearing.

As in all direct anterior approaches to the hip, the physical therapist should avoid straight leg raise exercises to avoid irritation of the iliopsoas tendon. No specific hip precautions are used.

OPEN REDUCTION AND INTERNAL FIXATION PLUS CONCOMITANT TOTAL HIP ARTHROPLASTY THROUGH A KOCHER-LANGENBECK APPROACH

If the primary acetabular fracture displacement is posterior, then consideration should be given to using the Kocher-Langenbeck approach for treatment. Posterior column, transverse, transverse-posterior wall, posterior column-posterior wall, and T-type fractures often fit this description. One relative contraindication to the use of this approach is central protrusion where the AIIS is comminuted or markedly displaced. Using a posterior approach in this situation may prove challenging because it is more difficult to reconstruct the AIIS from a Kocher-Langenbeck approach. In these cases, the Levine (anterior) approach to the hip as described above may be more suitable. Additionally, some patients who have sustained side impact trauma may have abrasions over the lateral aspect of the hip, which may preclude a Kocher-Langenbeck approach to the acetabulum. The advantages of this approach include its familiarity to both orthopedic trauma and joint replacement specialists and the speed at which the approach and reduction can be accomplished.

Surgical Technique

The patient is positioned in the lateral decubitus position usually on a radiolucent table (**Fig. 12**). Hip positioners are used to secure the patient, but fluoroscopy is used to make sure they do not obstruct fluoroscopic assessment of the acetabulum. The iliac oblique view is particularly susceptible to interference from positioners.

We use a typical Kocher-Langenbeck approach to the acetabulum. To protect the

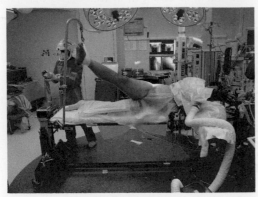

Fig. 12. For combined ORIF + THA through a Kocher-Langenbeck incision, the patient is positioned in a lateral decubitus position with the operative leg draped free. Standard THA positioners can be used, but care should be taken to make sure that they do not interfere with the fluoroscopy of the posterior column during the procedure. (*Courtesy of* T. Manson, MD, Baltimore, MD.)

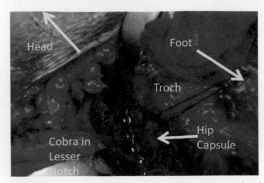

Fig. 13. In this image of a Kocher-Langenbeck approach to the acetabulum, the patient's head is off to the left and the foot off to the right. The posterior wall and column plates and screws are contoured directly over the capsule of the hip. This tethers the acetabular side of the hip capsule for secure capsular closure. (*Courtesy of* T. Manson, MD, Baltimore, MD.)

sciatic nerve, we do release the gluteus maximus sling for later repair[26] and we do keep the hip extended and knee flexed whenever instrumenting the posterior column. We do not typically use any neurologic monitoring. The acetabulum can be reconstructed with the femoral head in place as a template or with the femoral head removed to facilitate acetabular column reduction.

Acetabular reduction and fixation with the femoral head in place

With this strategy, we release the external rotators alone and tag them while leaving the capsule attached to the posterior trochanteric and acetabular wall and column fragments. We then reduce the posterior column fracture using Weber, Farabeuf, or Jungbluth clamps depending on fracture severity. Markedly comminuted posterior column fractures may benefit from multiple 2.7-mm reconstruction plates to reestablish native anatomy.

The posterior wall and column plates are placed directly over top of the hip capsule and therefore serve to tether the acetabular end of the hip capsule (Fig. 13). In this strategy, after fixation of the acetabulum, a separate sequential capsulotomy could then be made to dislocate the hip and resect the femoral head and neck. This step ensures that a roughly hemispherical acetabular fossa is recreated using the femoral head as a template. We typically use a 2.7- or 3.5-mm reconstruction plate to reconstruct the posterior column and then a 3.5-mm reconstruction plate used to reconstruct the posterior wall (Fig. 14).

Acetabular reduction and fixation after removing the femoral head

Another strategy is opening the capsule and resecting the femoral head before reduction and fixation of the acetabular fracture. Although this takes medially directed pressure off of the acetabulum, this strategy makes it easier to malreduce the acetabulum into an elliptical rather than hemispherical shape. Placing the resected femoral head (or a bipolar head trial) in the acetabulum every so often may help to avoid this end malreduction.

Acetabular reaming after fracture reduction

The femur is prepared using a standard femoral broaching technique and then attention is turned to the acetabulum. A large curved retractor with its spike into the region of the AIIS is used to retract the femur anteriorly to expose the acetabulum.

If the femur is difficult to retract anteriorly, then release of the head of the reflected rectus tendon just above the ilium usually allows anterior femoral translation. The direct head of the rectus is always left intact in this approach.

The labrum and pulvinar are resected. However, the transverse acetabular ligament is preserved because it is very helpful in acetabular component positioning.

We usually ream into the base of the cotyloid fossa first and then ream in sequential 2-mm increments up to the templated size.

We aim for a 1-mm press-fit. A standard multihole highly porous-coated revision acetabular

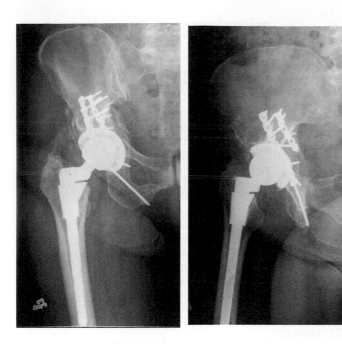

Fig. 14. This elderly patient had a comminuted posterior column and wall acetabular fracture that was treated with ORIF + THA through a Kocher-Langenbeck approach. The posterior column and wall were stabilized with a 2.7-mm reconstruction plate medially and 3.5-mm reconstruction plate laterally. (*Courtesy of* T. Manson, MD, Baltimore, MD.)

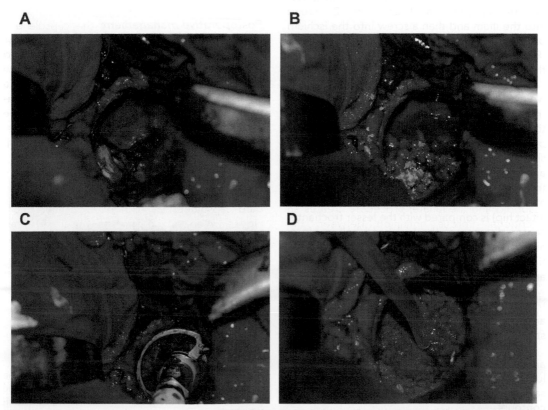

Fig. 15. (*A*) This image details a typical cavitary defect encountered when placing total hip replacements for acetabular fractures. The author typically uses impaction autograft to manage these defects. (*B*) The native femoral head is divided into 3 different sizes of particulate graft. Having 3 different particle sizes maximizes the structural and biological incorporation properties of the graft. (*C*) The author uses a reamer to reverse ream the graft into the defect. (*D*) This creates a stable medial bed to help resist medial protrusion of the acetabular component and also to reconstitute medial bone stock. (*Courtesy of* T. Manson, MD, Baltimore, MD.)

component is used. With this approach, we usually use the transverse acetabular ligament as well as fluoroscopy to guide component placement.

To mitigate against posterior dislocation we antevert the acetabular component slightly more than we would for THA for osteoarthritis (5° more anteversion). We also on average use larger femoral heads than we would in a case of primary THA for osteoarthritis. Higher dislocation results have been reported in the combined hip procedure and the increased anteversion and increased femoral head size are an attempt to minimize the occurrence of this complication.[8,11]

Large bony defects are treated with impaction grafting by morselizing the femoral head and reverse reaming of the morselized femoral head fragments into the acetabular fossa (Fig. 15).

We do place several supplemental bone screws and one of the chief challenges with this technique is finding screw corridors with the other posterior fixation implants in place. We usually place at least 1 or 2 screws into the ilium and then a screw into the ischium below the equator of the acetabular component (Fig. 16). We also sometimes place screws into the quadrilateral surface directly medially.

After fixation of the acetabulum using screws, we usually place a trial acetabular liner and test the stability of the hip. Usually, the hip is relatively stable. The combined version of the components should be around 40° and the hip should not dislocate with a position of flexion and deep adduction.[27–29] The lesser trochanter to center distance (as measured off the preoperative templated radiographs of the contralateral intact hip) is compared with the lesser trochanter center distance of the trial head ball in place, and this is the main judge of leg length recreation. Because the intact normal femoral head and neck are usually present during approach, we also record the native in situ lesser trochanter to center distance on the native femoral head and use this for comparison to our final reconstruction as well.

Usually, fluoroscopic images including and anteroposterior and Judet views of the acetabulum are used to make sure that the screws are in safe positions and not extending out of the bony contours.

The external rotators and hip capsule are closed using No. 5 Ethibond to the trailing edge of the gluteus medius (Fig. 17).[30–32] The gluteus maximus sling is closed using 0-PDS suture. The fascia lata is closed over an 1/8-inch

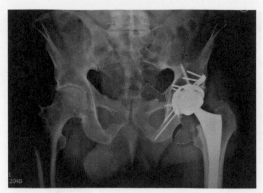

Fig. 16. Postoperative anteroposterior pelvis showing a patient was treated with concomitant ORIF + THA. Notice that screws have been placed superior into the ilium (*thin arrow*) and inferiorly into the ischium and ischial spine (*thick arrow*). This minimizes the tendency of the acetabular component to fail through abduction failure (*curved arrow*). (*Courtesy of* T. Manson, MD, Baltimore, MD.)

Hemovac drain and the skin closed using the surgeon's skin closure of choice.

Postoperative management

Patients are kept toe-touch weight bearing for 3 months postoperatively and then advanced slowly to weight bearing as tolerated with gradual relinquishment of assistant devices. We do use posterior hip precautions in these patients. Earlier weight bearing can probably be used depending on the displacement and overall comminution present in the posterior column.

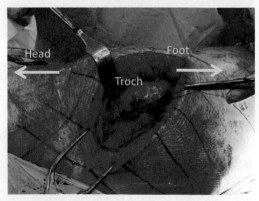

Fig. 17. At the conclusion of the procedure, the external rotators and hip capsule are repaired to the posterior edge of the gluteus medius with No. 5 Ethibond sutures. Alternatively, drill holes through the trochanter can also be used; however, for both primary and complex posterior hip replacement, the author's preference is for a dynamic repair to the trailing edge of the gluteus medius. (*Courtesy of* T. Manson, MD, Baltimore, MD.)

However in our center we have not moved to the use of earlier weight bearing.

ACKNOWLEDGMENTS

The author would like to thank Robert V. O'Toole III, MD, Marcus F. Sciadini, MD, and Jason W. Nascone, MD, for encouraging him to pursue the combined ORIF + THA for older patients with acetabular fractures. Their encouragement and critical questions spurred the development of the technique algorithms presented here.

REFERENCES

1. Matta JM. Fractures of the acetabulum: accuracy of reduction and clinical results in patients managed operatively within three weeks after the injury. J Bone Joint Surg Am 1996;78(11):1632–45.
2. Tannast M, Najibi S, Matta JM. Two to twenty year survivorship of the hip in 810 patients with operatively treated acetabular fractures. J Bone Joint Surg Am 2012;94(17):1559–67.
3. Anglen JO, Burd TA, Hendricks KJ, et al. The "gull sign": a harbinger of failure of internal fixation of geriatric acetabular fractures. J Orthop Trauma 2003;17(9):625–34.
4. Helfet DL, Borrelli J Jr, DiPasquale T, et al. Stabilization of acetabular fractures in elderly patients. J Bone Joint Surg Am 1992;74:753–65.
5. O'Toole RV, Hui E, Chandra A, et al. How often does open reduction and internal fixation of geriatric acetabular fractures lead to hip arthroplasty? J Orthop Trauma 2014;28:148–53.
6. Kreder HJ, Rozen N, Borkhoff CM, et al. Determinants of functional outcome after simple and complex acetabular fractures involving the posterior wall. J Bone Joint Surg Br 2006;88(6):776–82.
7. Beaulé PE, Griffin DB, Matta JM. The Levine anterior approach for total hip replacement as the treatment for an acute acetabular fracture. J Orthop Trauma 2004;18(9):623–9.
8. Boraiah S, Ragsdale M, Achor T, et al. Open reduction internal fixation and primary total hip arthroplasty of selected acetabular fractures. J Orthop Trauma 2009;23(4):243–8.
9. Chakravarty R, Toossi N, Katsman A, et al. Percutaneous column fixation and total hip arthroplasty for the treatment of acute acetabular fracture in the elderly. J Arthroplasty 2014;29(4):817–21.
10. Enocson A, Blomfeldt R. Acetabular fractures in the elderly treated with a primary Burch-Schneider reinforcement ring, autologous bone graft, and a total hip arthroplasty: a prospective study with a 4-year follow-up. J Orthop Trauma 2014;28(6):330–7.
11. Herscovici D, Lindvall E, Bolhofner B, et al. The combined hip procedure: open reduction internal fixation combined with total hip arthroplasty for the management of acetabular fractures in the elderly. J Orthop Trauma 2010;24(5):291–6.
12. Lin C, Caron J, Schmidt AH, et al. Functional outcomes after total hip arthroplasty for the acute management of acetabular fractures: 1-to 14-year follow-up. J Orthop Trauma 2015;29(3):151–9.
13. Malhotra R, Singh DP, Jain V, et al. Acute total hip arthroplasty in acetabular fractures in the elderly using the Octopus System: mid term to long term follow-up. J Arthroplasty 2013;28(6):1005–9.
14. Mears DC, Shirahama M. Stabilization of an acetabular fracture with cables for acute total hip arthroplasty. J Arthroplasty 1998;13(1):104–7.
15. Mears DC, Velyvis JH. Acute total hip arthroplasty for selected displaced acetabular fractures: two to twelve-year results. J Bone Joint Surg Am 2002; 84-A(1):1–9.
16. Mouhsine E, Garofalo R, Borens O, et al. Cable fixation and early total hip arthroplasty in the treatment of acetabular fractures in elderly patients. J Arthroplasty 2004;19(3):344–8.
17. Rickman M, Young J, Trompeter A, et al. Managing acetabular fractures in the elderly with fixation and primary arthroplasty: aiming for early weightbearing. Clin Orthop Relat Res 2014;472(11):3375–82.
18. Sermon A, Broos P, Vanderschot P. Total Hip replacement for acetabular fractures. Results in 121 patients operated on between 1983 and 2003. Injury 2008;39(8):914–21.
19. Tidermark J, Blomfeldt R, Ponzer S, et al. Primary total hip arthroplasty with a Burch-Schneider antiprotrusion cage and autologous bone grafting for acetabular fractures in elderly patients. J Orthop Trauma 2003;17(3):193–7.
20. Manson TT, O'Toole RV. ORIF vs arthroplasty of geriatric acetabular fractures: results of a randomized controlled feasibility study. Orthopaedic Trauma Association Annual Meeting. San Diego, California, October 7–11, 2015.
21. Sheth D, Cafri G, Inacio MC, et al. Anterior and anterolateral approaches for THA are associated with lower dislocation risk without higher revision risk. Clin Orthop Relat Res 2015;473(11): 3401–8.
22. Matta JM, Shahrdar C, Ferguson T. Single-incision anterior approach for total hip arthroplasty on an orthopaedic table. Clin Orthop Relat Res 2005; 441:115–24.
23. Surace P, Sultan AA, George J, et al. The association between operative time and short-term complications in total hip arthroplasty: an analysis of 89,802 surgeries. J Arthroplasty 2019; 34(3):426–32.
24. Wang Q, Goswami K, Shohat N, et al. Longer operative time results in a higher rate of subsequent periprosthetic joint infection in

patients undergoing primary joint arthroplasty. J Arthroplasty 2019;34(5):947–53.

25. Levine MA. A treatment of central fractures of the acetabulum. A case Report. J Bone Joint Surg 1943;25A:902–6.

26. Hurd JL, Potter HG, Dua V, et al. Sciatic nerve palsy after primary total hip arthroplasty: a new perspective. J Arthroplasty 2006;21(6): 796–802.

27. Dorr LD, Malik A, Dastane M, et al. Combined ante-version technique for total hip arthroplasty. Clin Orthop Relat Res 2009;467(1):119–27.

28. Lum ZC, Dorr LD. Restoration of center of rotation and balance of THR. J Orthop 2018;15(4):992–6.

29. Ranawat CS, Maynard MJ. Modern techniques of cemented total hip arthroplasty. Tech Orthop 1991;(6):17–25.

30. McLawhorn AS, Potter HG, Cross MB, et al. Poste-rior soft tissue repair after primary THA is durable at mid-term followup: a prospective MRI study. Clin Orthop Relat Res 2015;473(10):3183–9.

31. Pellicci PM, Bostrom M, Poss R. Posterior approach to total hip replacement using enhanced posterior soft tissue repair. Clin Orthop Relat Res 1998;355: 224–8.

32. Su EP, Mahoney CR, Adler RS, et al. Integrity of repaired posterior structures after THA. Clin Orthop Relat Res 2006;447:43–7.

Acute Distal Femoral Replacement for Fractures About the Knee in the Elderly

Olivia M. Rice, MD[a], Bryan D. Springer, MD[b],
Madhav A. Karunakar, MD[a],*

KEYWORDS

- Elderly • Distal femur fracture • Replantation • Distal femoral replacement • Megaprosthesis

---

KEY POINTS

- Distal femoral replacement is a reasonable treatment option for comminuted, intraarticular distal femur fractures in low-demand patients with poor bone quality.
- Indications for treatment with distal femoral replacement in the setting of acute distal femur fracture include the following:
  - Advanced age and low-demand functional status.
  - Multifragmentary, complete articular fractures (AO/OTA 33C) with evidence of "poor bone stock."
- Modern distal femoral replacement implants show favorable survivorship with minimal radiographic evidence of loosening.

INTRODUCTION: NATURE OF THE PROBLEM

Operative fixation of distal femur fractures (DFF) in osteoporotic bone is difficult.

These patients are often elderly and medically complex. Common fixation strategies often prohibit early ambulation, which may compromise clinical outcomes.[1] Similar to geriatric hip fractures, the risk of perioperative complications and mortality is high.[2] The use of distal femoral replacement (DFR) for acute DFF is rare, but published series suggest it may be a reasonable option in elderly patients.[3–10]

This article summarizes the existing literature on DFR for acute DFF in the elderly (Table 1). DFF of the native knee is the primary indication reviewed. DFR literature for periprosthetic fractures (PPF) exist elsewhere,[11–18] but variations in treatment strategy relative to indication are compared throughout.

TERMINOLOGY
Distal Femoral Replacement

- A rotating hinge prosthesis that replaces a "large" segment of the distal femur. No standard definition exists detailing the amount of femoral bone resected. Generally, the distal femoral resection is proximal to the insertion of the knee's collateral ligaments.[a]
- This definition does *not* include use of a rotating hinge prosthesis for surface

---

Disclosure Statement: B.D. Springer: Consultant for Stryker/ConvaTec; Receives royalties from Stryker; Board member of Knee Society, AJRR, and ICJR; Medical advisor for Joint Purification Solutions. The remaining authors have nothing to disclose.

[a] Department of Orthopaedic Surgery, Carolinas Medical Center, Atrium Health Musculoskeletal Institute, 1025 Morehead Medical Drive, Suite 300, Charlotte, NC 28204, USA; [b] OrthoCarolina Hip and Knee Center, Atrium Health Musculoskeletal Institute, 2001 Vail Avenue Suite 200A, Charlotte, NC 28207, USA
* Corresponding author.
E-mail address: madhav.karunakar@atriumhealth.org

[a]Authors' opinion and/or experience.

Table 1
Study characteristics of literature reporting distal femoral replacement use for acute distal femur fractures in the elderly

Author, Year	N	Avg Age in y [Range]	Study Type	Level of Evidence
Appleton et al,[3] 2006	54	82 [55–98]	Retrospective Case Series	Level IV
Atrey et al,[4] 2017	4	74 [52–102]	Retrospective Case Series	Level IV
Bettin et al,[5] 2016	18	77 [62–94]	Retrospective Case Series	Level IV
Hart et al,[6] 2017	10	82 [71–92]	Retrospective Cohort	Level III
Neal et al,[7] 2019	1	80	Case Report	Level IV
Pearse et al,[8] 2005	6	85 [77–94]	Retrospective Cohort	Level III
Totals	93	[a]80 [66–93]	- -	- -

Abbreviations: Avg, average; N, number of joints.
[a] Avg.

level replacement that may be used in complex primary or revision arthroplasty.

- Synonyms of DFR include "megaprosthesis" and "endoprosthesis." All DFR implants in the literature were previously reviewed.[18]

Acute

- Treated within 1 month of injury

As opposed to a fracture nonunion due to failed management of another cause.

Native Knee

- Without existing hardware

Referring to the absence of a total knee arthroplasty (TKA) implant. This definition includes knees operated on for other reasons besides TKA, without residual hardware.

INDICATIONS AND CONTRAINDICATIONS FOR USE

The most common indications and contraindications for DFR in acute DFF are listed in **Tables 2** and **3**, respectively. Kuzyk and colleagues describe the indication for revision arthroplasty in the setting of periprosthetic DFF as those "associated with loose or malaligned implants, with or without severe bone loss." Specifically, DFR is indicated when the "bone is too comminuted or too distal for standard revision TKA, or in which bone stock prevents acceptable fixation techniques."

Nontraumatic DFR indications include the following:

- Oncologic reconstruction for distal femur tumors[19]
- Primary complex TKA[20]

- Revision TKA[21]
  - Including for infection via a 2-stage procedure

An important factor *not* listed in the contraindications from prior literature is *open* fractures. Multiple published studies analyzing native and periprosthetic DFF included open fractures in their analysis.[5,7,22] No studies listed it as a contraindication to DFR use. Patients with

Table 2
Indications most commonly found in the literature with a brief description

Indication	Comments
Fracture pattern AO/OTA 33C[48]	Complex intraarticular extension limits option of retrograde nail[26] Anatomic reduction and stable fixation with a locking plate limited by comminution close to the joint line (small distal segment)[26]
Poor bone stock[4,15,22,33,49]	Osteoporotic bone proximal to the fracture cannot tolerate the forces of a rigid fixation construct
Advanced age	Unable to tolerate partial weight-bearing postop[6] Prevent complications of immobility[4] Eliminate risk for nonunion[26]
Ipsilateral knee OA[3,4,14] or rheumatoid arthritis[27,33,50]	OA severity determined via plain radiographs showing subchondral sclerosis or cysts and periarticular osteophytes[5]

Abbreviation: OA, osteoarthritis.

Table 3
Contraindications most commonly found in the literature with a brief description

Contraindication	Comments
Young age/active	Bone amenable to alternative modes of fixation Longevity of patient > implant[9]
Active infection[10]	Eradicate infection before arthroplasty Alternative: 2-stage procedure[14] OR silver-coated DFR[19]
Ipsilateral long-stem hip implant	Risk of interprosthetic fracture Alternative: custom-made "linked" prosthesis[51]
Disrupted extensor mechanism	Tension required for appropriate implant stability[4]
Nonambulatory status	Unable to benefit from early weight-bearing[10]

open injuries underwent surgery for formal irrigation and debridement within 24 hours of presentation.[5,7] Bettin and colleagues[5] resected the DFF at this time and placed an antibiotic spacer as well. Subsequently, patients returned to the OR within a few days for definitive treatment with DFR.[7]

For each patient, the potential benefits of arthroplasty surgery are compared against their baseline ambulatory status and overall health. This decision often involves a goal-of-care discussion with the patient and their family.

Important patient history components include the following:

- Age
  - No "cutoff" age currently exists. Various studies use arbitrary ages for inclusion criteria,[3–6] ranging from 50 to 75 years old, ultimately determined by surgeon preference.
  - Clement and colleagues states, "the longevity of the patient should probably not be longer than that of the implant."
- Medical comorbidities
  - Ability to tolerate the physiologic insult of surgery
  - Ability to partially weight-bear if necessary, that is, cognitive function
  - Risk factors associated with fragility fractures (Fracture Risk Assessment Tool score)[23]
- Preoperative ambulatory status
- Preinjury visits to an orthopedic arthroplasty surgeon (preexisting OA)

PREOPERATIVE CARE
Logistics
Orthopedic surgeons from multiple subspecialties have previously reported their experience with DFR use for various nontumor indications.[5,19,24] The general recommendation surrounds DFR use in the hands of a surgeon familiar and comfortable with the implant, without explicitly noting a subspecialty most suited for it.

However, if the admitting surgeon is NOT the treating surgeon[a], transferring the patient's care may require teamwork. Similar to the hip fracture cohort, assistance from comanagement teams (eg, geriatric or internal medicine physicians) likely improves patient outcomes.[25]

Timing of Surgery
The patient should be medically optimized before surgery. Additional days in the hospital before definitive fixation compared with those treated with ORIF may occur for several reasons:

- Patients indicated for DFR are generally older with more medical comorbidities. Therefore, aggressive optimization and extended time before clearance for surgery may be necessary.[5]
- Care coordination, as mentioned earlier, may include physically transferring the patient to another hospital location[a].
- Order and shipment of specialty implants not otherwise kept in stock.
- Use of custom DFR implants that require patient-specific templating and manufacturing.

Provisional Reduction
Closed reduction and immobilization with a long leg splint or knee immobilizer should be performed on initial presentation until time of surgery.

Imaging and Preoperative Planning
- Computed tomography (CT) +/− 3-dimensional reconstruction

o Preoperative CT scans of DFF are often obtained in the era of low-dose radiation machines.[a] They supplement the decision-making process for treatment strategy and assist in preoperative planning. A common rationale for obtaining a CT scan for a DFF includes the following:
  ▪ Evaluate the amount of bone available for fixation
  ▪ Identify coronal plane fractures
  ▪ In the setting of PPF, determine the stability of the implant
o CT scans can also provide valuable information for assessing the length, alignment, and rotation intraoperatively. According to Kuzyk and colleagues, a scan of the "bilateral hips and knees gives the most accurate estimation of lower extremity rotation, assuming the contralateral knee is intact."
- Plain radiographs of injured extremity plus joints above and below
o To identify other injuries plus preexisting prostheses, especially in the ipsilateral hip[26]
- Plain radiographs of the contralateral extremity, if intact
o To use for implant templating[27]
o To assess for leg length discrepancy; if present, a unique opportunity exists to fix it concurrently[15]

Soft Tissue Assessment

- Evaluate skin for preexisting scars, wounds from injury, and soft tissue envelope[26]
- Consult plastic surgery for assistance with soft tissue coverage, if necessary[26]

INTRAOPERATIVE TECHNIQUE
Common Themes

- Perioperative antibiotics[3–8]
o Generally, follow standard total joint arthroplasty antibiotic prophylaxis
- Tourniquet[3–5,7,8]
o Sterile or nonsterile depending on proximal extent of femoral fixation
- Anatomic approach (using previous scars if applicable)
o Skin incision: anterior, midline, longitudinal/extensile
o Arthrotomy: medial parapatellar
- Fracture fixation
o Resection

▪ Bone and soft tissue attachments removed within the fracture site
o Some prefer to use an osteotome or oscillating saw to resect slightly proximal to the fracture.[15,17]
o Cerclage wires or cables for reinforcement of fixation due to proximal extension of the fracture line or osteopenia are also described.[7,22]

Implant Choice
Many brands of modular hinge prostheses exist on the market.[21] Choice is based on surgeon preference or institutional availability. Please see **Box 1** for examples of DFR implants previously published for use in acute DFF.

Implant Augments

- Cement
  Generally, both tibial and femoral stems are cemented for elderly patients with osteoporotic bone. However, some studies show cement increases rates of aseptic loosening.[28] Its use with surface type hinged prostheses for nontraumatic indications declined when metaphyseal cones arrived; however, it is still commonly used for DFR in acute fracture indications.[13,15]
  Depending on surgeon preference and patient bone quality, options for stem fixation include the following:
  o Cemented stem fixation[3,4,7,8]
  o Press fit (cementless fixation)
  o Some opt to infuse the cement with antibiotics[5,7] for periprosthetic joint infection prophylaxis; albeit its efficacy is controversial.[a]

Box 1
Distal femoral replacement prostheses reported in the literature for the indication of acute distal femur fracture

Stanmore Hinge Prosthesis (Zimmer-Biomet, Warsaw, IN)

Orthopedic Salvage System (Biomet, Warsaw, IN)

Global Segmental System Distal Femur (Zimmer, Warsaw, IN)

Modular Replacement System (Stryker, Mahwah, NJ)

- Allograft
  - Nonstructural, that is, cancellous bone chips[29]
  - Structural[15]
- Metaphyseal sleeves
  - Designed to augment contained bone defects in the distal femoral metaphysis and proximal tibia; commonly used in primary and revision TKA. It is less commonly for DFR in acute fracture, as the femoral resection is typically above the level of the metaphysis. However, a sleeve may be used in the tibia if necessary.[14,15,17,29]
- Hydroxyapatite-coated collar[30]
  - Creates biologic ingrowth at the proximal femoral bony interface[31]
- Silver-coated implant[19] (included for completeness)
  - May decrease risk of deep infection in high-risk patients[32]
  - Perhaps not applicable for acute DFF but can be considered in a patient at high risk for infection (eg, recent history of systemic sepsis or history of infected hardware removal)
- Patella
  - Replaced, resurfaced, or left alone, according to surgeon preference[33,34]
  - It may be reasonable to resurface if chondral disease is present[10]

POSTOPERATIVE CARE
Weight-Bearing Status

- Weight-bearing as tolerated to bilateral lower extremities following surgery, when possible, is unanimous in the literature[3–8]

Prophylaxis

- Antibiotics
  - Some report using a "standard post-TKA protocol" including prophylactic antibiotics for several days postoperatively
- Venous thromboembolism
  - Universally reported, most did not specify type or duration
  - Surgeon and institution preference

Rehabilitation

- Physical therapy (PT)
  - Included in some "post-TKA'" protocols; some inpatients working with PT twice daily[5]
  - Surgeon and institution preference

OUTCOMES

Many reviews and retrospective case-series describe DFR use for various indications. Unfortunately, most data are reported in a way that prevents separation of the outcomes by indication.[9,10] Definitions of postoperative complications are variable, prohibiting clean data comparison.

Six studies (93 patients) were identified in literature published in the past 15 years.[3–8] Other published DFR studies included patients with acute DFF[9,10,35,36]; however, the outcome and demographic data could not be isolated and therefore are not included in Table 4.

Functional Outcomes

- The most commonly reported functional outcome measure was knee range of motion (ROM). Three of the reviewed

Table 4
Complications with distal femoral replacement for acute distal femur fracture

Author	LOS	Reoperation	Implant Revision	Deep Infection	PPF	Mortality (1 y)
Appleton et al,[3] 2006	15 [12–23]	7	3	1	4	22
Atrey et al,[4] 2017	26 [15–56]	0	0	0	0	0
Bettin et al,[5] 2016	11 [5–43]	4	2	1	1	1
Hart et al,[6] 2017	7 [4–12]	1	0	1	0	1
Neal et al,[7] 2019	12	0	0	0	0	0
Pearse et al,[8] 2005	15 [9–19][b]	0	0	0	0	0
Totals (%)	[a]14 [9–19]	12 (13%)	5 (5%)	3 (3%)	5 (5%)	24 (26%)

Abbreviations: Avg, average; LOS, length of stay; PPF, periprosthetic fracture.
[a] Avg.
[b] Postop days only.

studies[5,7,8] included this metric, with average postoperative ROM = 0° to 98°.

Complications

- PPF was the most common surgical complication reported, followed by deep infection. These complications required reoperation in all cases and revision or removal of the implant in most circumstances. Three of the 4 PPF reported by Appleton and colleagues[3] were interprosthetic fractures that occurred between the DFR implant and a hip prosthesis.
- Other complications included superficial infection treated with oral antibiotics.[5,6]
- The overall mortality rate at 1 year was 26%. Appleton and colleagues[3] reported most of these deaths, likely due to the significant comorbidities associated with their patient cohort. They included many nonambulatory patients and others with cognitive impairment or who are socially dependent. However, this is the most extensive case series using DFR for acute DFF reported to date.

A summary of the data reported on complications and other standard hospital metrics can be found in **Table 4**.

The historically high incidence of aseptic loosening is often quoted as a reason to avoid DFR use.[3,36] There were no patients in this review with evidence of aseptic loosening, with average follow-up of 3 years. Authors of the revision TKA literature hypothesize that the advent of metaphyseal sleeves dramatically decreases the risk of this problem.[29] However, it is unclear how common the use of these sleeves is for DFR use in acute fracture.

Limitations
Inconsistent reporting methods

- Surgical technique, including the type of prosthesis
  DFR, megaprosthesis, endoprosthesis, and rotating hinged-knee prosthesis are often used interchangeably. Important details commonly missing include the following:
  - Name or type of implants used for the femur and/or tibia
  - Amount of distal femur resected (or if it was resected)
  - Types of augmentation used

- Outcomes
  - Different metrics and functional outcomes are reported throughout the literature. One example is "length of stay." Some studies only report postoperative days in hospital.[8] Others report total inpatient days, which may or may not include time spent in an inpatient rehabilitation unit.[3,4,6] The "length of stay" metric influences the total cost of the inpatient stay, which is critical for economic analysis. These details are minor, but over time, it limits the ability to congregate data for meta-analysis.

Comparisons of Distal Femoral Replacement Outcomes Stratified by Indication

Many articles describe DFR use in revision TKA[14,15,21,24,33,37–44] as well, gaining popularity for the treatment of PPF in particular.[13–15,24,37,41–44] The inability to differentiate outcomes based on indication is often referenced as a "weakness" of published data. However, it is unclear whether differences in DFR outcomes for nononcologic indications exist.

The following 2 studies[9,45] assessed differences between cohorts separated by indication:

- Primary TKA with DFR following periprosthetic DFF (n = 36) versus conversion to DFR after failed ORIF of periprosthetic DFF (n = 13)
  - There were no significant differences in outcomes.[45]
- DFR for acute DFF versus DFR for revision arthroplasty for any reason:
  - Hospital length of stay (LOS) and likelihood to discharge to a higher dependency of care were higher in the acute DFF cohort.
  - There were no significant differences in mortality, reoperation, or other complications.[9]

Direct comparisons between DFR outcomes lack convincing evidence. However, Streubel and colleagues recently compared mortality rates following distal (native and periprosthetic) and proximal femur fractures. PPF and higher age-adjusted Charlson comorbidity index[46] were associated with decreased survival (HR = 3.21, P = .005 and HR = 1.32, P = .004, respectively). They also showed that patients whose surgery occurred 4 or more days after injury versus before 48 hours from injury had significantly increased 6-month and 1-year mortality risks. The underlying factors behind these outcomes are unknown; however, other investigators have failed to reproduce similar results.[5,22]

FUTURE WORK
Economic Cost Analysis
The substantial cost of a DFR implant is a conventional deterrent to its use. Many argue that after implant cost is combined into the total cost of care, the cost difference between implants is negligible.[6,8] Others report potential for a decreased number of total lifetime procedures and shorter LOS (rehab facility LOS included)[22] with DFR.

However, these claims have yet to be proved. A postinjury "lifetime" cost comparison between

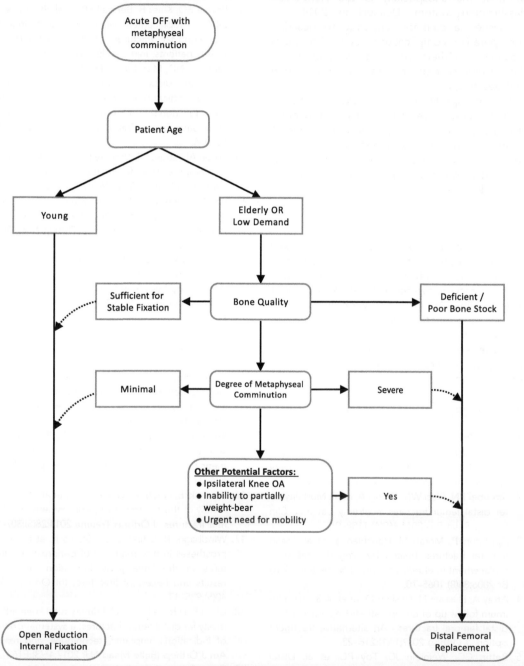

Fig. 1. Indications for DFR—patient treatment algorithm. Solid arrows represent common indications. Dotted arrows represent relative indications that are patient specific and depend on surgeon preference. Operative Reduction Internal Fixation includes retrograde femoral nail. OA, osteoarthritis.

different treatment modalities of acute DFF in the elderly may settle this debate.

Reporting Standards and Comparison of Patient Cohorts

Most of the literature describing DFR use is for oncologic reconstruction, which was DFR's primary indication. A standard outcome metric amongst the subspecialty is the Henderson classification system. Defined in 2014,[47] it established a common language to describe postoperative complications seen with endoprostheses. Others suggested adopting this classification schema universally when reporting DFR outcomes.[39]

The orthopedic literature uses inconsistent terminology when referencing distal femoral replacements and their respective indications. A common language to communicate the indications and outcomes of DFR use is necessary for systematic reviews and is essential for research moving forward.

SUMMARY

DFR is a reasonable treatment option when used for select indications (see **Table 2**). In the setting of a comminuted intraarticular DFF, DFR should be considered in low-demand patients with poor bone quality. An institution-wide initiative to support coordination between subspecialties may be helpful.

Please see **Fig. 1** for an algorithm to decipher which patients are most appropriate for DFR consideration.

REFERENCES

1. Liu VX, Rosas E, Hwang J, et al. Enhanced recovery after surgery program implementation in 2 surgical populations in an integrated health care delivery system. JAMA Surg 2017;152(7):e171032.
2. Streubel PN, Ricci WM, Wong A, et al. Mortality after distal femur fractures in elderly patients. Clin Orthop Relat Res 2011;469(4):1188–96.
3. Appleton P, Moran M, Houshian S, et al. Distal femoral fractures treated by hinged total knee replacement in elderly patients. J Bone Joint Surg Br 2006;88(8):1065–70.
4. Atrey A, Hussain N, Gosling O, et al. A 3 year minimum follow up of Endoprosthetic replacement for distal femoral fractures - An alternative treatment option. J Orthop 2017;14(1):216–22.
5. Bettin CC, Weinlein JC, Toy PC, et al. Distal femoral replacement for acute distal femoral fractures in elderly patients. J Orthop Trauma 2016; 30(9):503–9.
6. Hart GP, Kneisl JS, Springer BD, et al. Open reduction vs distal femoral replacement arthroplasty for comminuted distal femur fractures in the patients 70 years and older. J Arthroplasty 2017;32(1):202–6.
7. Neal DC, Sambhariya V, Tran A, et al. Single-stage bilateral distal femur replacement for traumatic distal femur fractures. Arthroplast Today 2019;5(1): 26–31.
8. Pearse EO, Klass B, Bendall SP, et al. Stanmore total knee replacement versus internal fixation for supracondylar fractures of the distal femur in elderly patients. Injury 2005;36(1):163–8.
9. Clement ND, MacDonald D, Moran M, et al. Mega prosthetic distal femoral arthroplasty for non-tumour indications: does the indication affect the functional outcome and survivorship? Knee Surg Sports Traumatol Arthrosc 2015;23(5): 1330–6.
10. Rosen AL, Strauss E. Primary total knee arthroplasty for complex distal femur fractures in elderly patients. Clin Orthop Relat Res 2004;425:101–5.
11. Ebraheim NA, Carroll T, Bonaventura B, et al. Challenge of managing distal femur fractures with long-stemmed total knee implants. Orthop Surg 2014; 6(3):217–22.
12. Herrera DA, Kregor PJ, Cole PA, et al. Treatment of acute distal femur fractures above a total knee arthroplasty: systematic review of 415 cases (1981-2006). Acta Orthop 2008;79(1):22–7.
13. Khan S, Schmidt AH. Distal femoral replacement for periprosthetic fractures around total knee arthroplasty: when and how? J Knee Surg 2019; 32(5):388–91.
14. Kouk S, Rathod PA, Maheshwari AV, et al. Rotating hinge prosthesis for complex revision total knee arthroplasty: a review of the literature. J Clin Orthop Trauma 2018;9(1):29–33.
15. Kuzyk PRT, Watts E, Backstein D. Revision total knee arthroplasty for the management of periprosthetic fractures. J Am Acad Orthop Surg 2017;25(9): 624–33.
16. Ristevski B, Nauth A, Williams DS, et al. Systematic review of the treatment of periprosthetic distal femur fractures. J Orthop Trauma 2014;28(5):307–12.
17. Windhager R, Schreiner M, Staats K, et al. Mega-prostheses in the treatment of periprosthetic fractures of the knee joint: indication, technique, results and review of literature. Int Orthop 2016; 40(5):935–43.
18. Chen F, Li R, Lall A, et al. Primary total knee arthroplasty for distal femur fractures: a systematic review of indications, implants, techniques, and results. Am J Orthop (Belle Mead NJ) 2017;46(3):E163–71.
19. Evans S, Laugharne E, Kotecha A, et al. Megaprostheses in the management of trauma of the knee. J Orthop 2016;13(4):467–71.

20. Gehrke T, Kendoff D, Haasper C. The role of hinges in primary total knee replacement. Bone Joint J 2014;96B(11):93–5.

21. Rodríguez-Merchán EC. Total knee arthroplasty using hinge joints: Indications and results. EFORT Open Rev 2019;4(4):121–32.

22. Hoellwarth JS, Fourman MS, Crossett L, et al. Equivalent mortality and complication rates following periprosthetic distal femur fractures managed with either lateral locked plating or a distal femoral replacement. Injury 2018;49(2):392–7.

23. Baim S, Leslie WD. Assessment of fracture risk. Curr Osteoporos Rep 2012;10(1):28–41.

24. Girgis E, McAllen C, Keenan J. Revision knee arthroplasty using a distal femoral replacement prosthesis for periprosthetic fractures in elderly patients. Eur J Orthop Surg Traumatol 2018;28(1):95–102.

25. Konda SR, Pean CA, Goch AM, et al. Comparison of short-term outcomes of geriatric distal femur and femoral neck fractures. Geriatr Orthop Surg Rehabil 2015;6(4):311–5.

26. Hake ME, Davis ME, Perdue AM, et al. Modern implant options for the treatment of distal femur fractures. J Am Acad Orthop Surg 2019. https://doi.org/10.5435/JAAOS-D-17-00706.

27. Donnelly KJ, Tucker A, Ruiz A, et al. Managing extremely distal periprosthetic femoral supracondylar fractures of total knee replacements - a new PHILOS-ophy. World J Orthop 2017;8(10):809–13.

28. Hu CC, Chen SY, Chen CC, et al. Superior survivorship of cementless vs cemented diaphyseal fixed modular rotating-hinged knee megaprosthesis at 7 years' follow-up. J Arthroplasty 2017;32(6):1940–5.

29. Cottino U, Abdel MP, Perry KI, et al. Long-term results after total knee arthroplasty with contemporary rotating-hinge prostheses. J Bone Joint Surg Am 2017;99(4):324–30.

30. Konan S, Sandiford N, Unno F, et al. Periprosthetic fractures associated with total knee arthroplasty an update. Bone Joint J 2016;98-B(11):1489–96.

31. Myers GJC, Abudu AT, Carter SR, et al. Endoprosthetic replacement of the distal femur for bone tumours: long- term results. J Bone Joint Surg Br 2007;89(4):521–6.

32. Gautam D, Malhotra R. Megaprosthesis versus allograft prosthesis composite for massive skeletal defects. J Clin Orthop Trauma 2018;9(1):63–80.

33. Efe T, Roessler PP, Heyse TJ, et al. Mid-term results after implantation of rotating-hinge knee prostheses: primary versus revision. Orthop Rev (Pavia) 2012;4(4):35.

34. Rao B, Kamal T, Vafe J, et al. Distal femoral replacement for selective periprosthetic fractures above a total knee arthroplasty. Eur J Trauma Emerg Surg 2014;40(2):191–9.

35. Springer BD, Hanssen AD, Sim FH, et al. The kinematic rotating hinge prosthesis for complex knee arthroplasty. Clin Orthop Relat Res 2001;392:283–91.

36. Berend KR, Lombardi AVJ. Distal femoral replacement in nontumor cases with severe bone loss and instability. Clin Orthop Relat Res 2009;467(2):485–92.

37. Saidi K, Ben-Lulu O, Tsuji M, et al. Supracondylar periprosthetic fractures of the knee in the elderly patients: a comparison of treatment using allograft-implant composites, standard revision components, distal femoral replacement prosthesis. J Arthroplasty 2014;29(1):110–4.

38. Springer BD, Sim FH, Hanssen AD, et al. The modular segmental kinematic rotating hinge for nonneoplastic limb salvage. Clin Orthop Relat Res 2004;421:181–7.

39. Toepfer A, Harrasser N, Schwarz PR, et al. Distal femoral replacement with the MML system: a single center experience with an average follow-up of 86 months. BMC Musculoskelet Disord 2017;18(1):1–7.

40. Harrison RJJ, Thacker MM, Pitcher JD, et al. Distal femur replacement is useful in complex total knee arthroplasty revisions. Clin Orthop Relat Res 2006;446:113–20.

41. Holl S, Schlomberg A, Gosheger G, et al. Distal femur and proximal tibia replacement with megaprosthesis in revision knee arthroplasty: a limb-saving procedure. Knee Surg Sports Traumatol Arthrosc 2012;20(12):2513–8.

42. Keenan J, Chakrabarty G, Newman JH. Treatment of supracondylar femoral fracture above total knee replacement by custom made hinged prosthesis. Knee 2000;7(3):165–70.

43. Pradhan NR, Bale L, Kay P, et al. Salvage revision total knee replacement using the Endo-Model® rotating hinge prosthesis. Knee 2004;11(6):469–73.

44. Rajgopal A, Vasdev A, Chidgupkar AS, et al. Mid-term results of rotating hinge knee prostheses. Acta Orthop Belg 2012;78(1):61–7.

45. Chen AF, Choi LE, Colman MW, et al. Primary versus secondary distal femoral arthroplasty for treatment of total knee arthroplasty periprosthetic femur fractures. J Arthroplasty 2013;28(9):1580–4.

46. Charlson M, Szatrowski TP, Peterson J, et al. Validation of a combined comorbidity index. J Clin Epidemiol 1994;47(11):1245–51.

47. Henderson ER, O'Connor MI, Ruggieri P, et al. Classification of failure of limb salvage after reconstructive surgery for bone tumours: a modified system including biological and expandable reconstructions. Bone Joint J 2014;96B(11):1436–40.

48. Kellam JF, Meinberg EG, Agel J, et al. AO/OTA fracture and dislocation classification compendium - 2018. J Orthop Trauma 2018;32S:40–3.

49. Ruder JA, Hart GP, Kneisl JS, et al. Predictors of functional recovery following periprosthetic distal femur fractures. J Arthroplasty 2017;32(5): 1571–5.

50. Mortazavi SMJ, Kurd MF, Bender B, et al. Distal femoral arthroplasty for the treatment of periprosthetic fractures after total knee arthroplasty. J Arthroplasty 2010;25(5):775–80.

51. Patel NK, Whittingham-Jones P, Aston WJ, et al. Custom-made cement-linked mega prostheses: a salvage solution for complex periprosthetic femoral fractures. J Arthroplasty 2014;29(1):204–9.

Pediatrics

Treatment for Post-Slipped Capital Femoral Epiphysis Deformity

Melissa M. Allen, MD, MSCR[a], Scott B. Rosenfeld, MD[b],*

KEYWORDS

- Slipped capital femoral epiphysis • Femoroacetabular impingement • Hip arthroscopy
- Surgical hip dislocation • Intertrochanteric osteotomy

KEY POINTS

- Slipped capital femoral epiphysis results in altered proximal femoral anatomy with variable remodeling potential that may produce femoroacetabular impingement.
- Femoroacetabular impingement has been shown to result in early intraarticular damage, reduced hip function, and an increased risk of premature arthritis.
- Hip arthroscopy is a good method for correcting mild deformities through osteochondroplasty and allows simultaneous treatment of labral and cartilage pathology.
- Moderate and severe deformities may require extensile exposure through a surgical hip dislocation approach, which allows global access to the femoral head–neck junction for open femoroplasty as well as to the acetabulum for treatment of intraarticular derangements.
- Intertrochanteric osteotomy is a powerful correction tool that can be used alone or in combination with open osteochondroplasty for reorientation of the femoral head and neck.

INTRODUCTION

Slipped capital femoral epiphysis (SCFE) is the most common adolescent hip disorder, and the incidence has risen with increasing obesity rates.[1] The primary goal of treatment is to stabilize the physis against further slippage and prevent it from becoming unstable, which is associated with an avascular necrosis rate of up to 47%.[2] Reports in the literature have shown that patients who develop avascular necrosis have poor outcomes, so any treatment modality must also minimize this complication.[3] Because reductive manipulation of the SCFE may lead to iatrogenic avascular necrosis, the current gold standard treatment modality is in situ pinning—regardless of the degree of deformity.[4] This technique may successfully stabilize

the physis, but does result in residual deformity of the proximal femur. Although a variable amount of remodeling is possible, many patients will have some amount of persistent residual changes in their proximal femoral anatomy. The short-term to midterm outcomes for these patients is generally good to excellent, even with a grade III slip.[5] However, longer term studies have highlighted lower activity scores and persistent pain in approximately one-third of patients. Larson and colleagues[6] performed a retrospective review of 176 hips at an average follow-up of 16 years. They reported that by 10 years after in situ pinning, 10.5% of patients had undergone a second surgery, including conversion to total hip arthroplasty. Seventeen percent of patients in that cohort had a fair or poor outcome.

Disclosure Statement: The authors have nothing to disclose.
a Pediatric Orthopedic Surgery, Baylor College of Medicine, 6701 Fannin Street, MWT 660.00, Houston, TX 77030, USA; b Pediatric Orthopedic Surgery, Baylor College of Medicine, Hip Preservation Center, Texas Children's Hospital, 6701 Fannin Street, MWT 660.00, Houston, TX 77030, USA
* Corresponding author.
E-mail address: sbrosenf@texaschildrens.org

With improved understanding of abnormal hip biomechanics,[7] as well as new surgical techniques, there is increased interest in identifying ways to improve long-term outcomes for patients with SCFE. In the last decade especially, the association between residual hip deformity after in situ pinning and symptomatic femoroacetabular impingement (FAI) has been identified as a potential cause for both short- and long-term hip dysfunction.[8] In the immediate time frame after an SCFE, FAI morphology can result in decreased hip range of motion, labral tears, and articular cartilage damage.[9]

There is a growing body of evidence to support that post-SCFE deformity, like idiopathic FAI, results in mechanical damage to the peripheral acetabular cartilage. Lee and colleagues[10] reviewed 5 patients with mild to moderate slips who underwent arthroscopy and femoral osteoplasty within 18 months after in situ stabilization and found all had gross labral and/or acetabular cartilage damage anterosuperiorly, which is the characteristic location for impingement related pathology.[7] In a multicenter review[11] of 109 patients who underwent surgical hip dislocations for realignment of slips of greater than 30°, 89% had cartilage damage ranging from an abrasion to full-thickness loss in the anterior superior quadrant. The amount of injury was independent of the slip severity or duration of symptoms before surgery.

In addition to the direct signs of pain, loss of motion, and abnormal gait, the cumulative damage from FAI is a risk factor for progression of osteoarthritis, even in the absence of symptoms for many years.[12] One study[8] of 121 SCFE patients treated by in situ pinning at a mean follow-up of 22 years found radiographic signs of FAI in 79% and osteoarthritis in all. The mean Harris Hip Score was significantly worse in the patients with FAI, and the degree of deformity was directly correlated with osteoarthritis in early adulthood. Another report[13] of 58 hips at 30 to 40 years of follow-up showed significantly worse outcomes for those with abnormal and higher alpha angles. In that cohort, 15% to 25% of patients with a mild slip had osteoarthritis. A separate radiographic study[14] found the final alpha angle after years of remodeling still averaged 66°. Even in the absence of symptoms, alpha angles of greater than 60° have been correlated with degenerative changes on delayed gadolinium-enhanced MRI of cartilage, which has been shown to be useful in detecting early arthrosis.[15] The findings of increased alpha angles and decreased head–neck offset in patients with SCFE is a separate type of deformity than that of the slip angle, and they are significantly altered even when the slip is mild.[16]

The risks of ongoing intraarticular damage secondary to post-SCFE deformity have prompted many surgeons to advocate for dedicated treatment of FAI morphology as a means of hip preservation.[17] Although techniques such as the modified Dunn procedure exist for immediate correction of SCFE deformity, most have not gained widespread acceptance owing to the increased risk profile and specialized training that are required compared with in situ pinning.[18] Fortunately, several techniques are available to correct residual deformity after initial physeal stabilization has been achieved.

PATHOLOGY

In an SCFE, the metaphysis translates anteriorly and externally rotates while the epiphysis remains in a relatively posterior position within the acetabulum (Fig. 1). The uncovered anterior and lateral metaphyseal corner may form a discrete prominence or bump that impinges against the labrum, the rim of the acetabulum, and the peripheral acetabular articular cartilage[19] (Fig. 2). Radiographically, the metaphyseal translation decreases the head–neck offset and increases the alpha angle. The change in epiphyseal–metaphyseal orientation also results in relative femoral retroversion and coxa vara in some cases.

The typical post-SCFE deformity has been described as a cam-type lesion, which has been further classified into inclusion or impaction as defined by Rab.[20] Inclusion is seen in mild slips and refers to a lesion that is small enough to

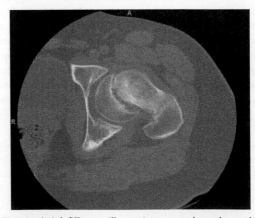

Fig. 1. Axial CT scan illustrating anterolateral translation of the metaphysis with relatively posterior positioning of the epiphysis.

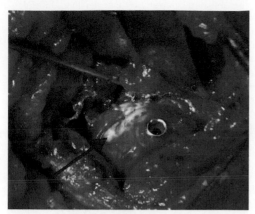

Fig. 2. View of a discrete metaphyseal-epiphyseal prominence (*arrow*) located adjacent to a torn labrum and just above the previously inserted SCFE screw.

enter into the joint, where it can compress and shear across the articular cartilage (**Fig. 3**). Over time, such a small metaphyseal prominence can remodel to become part of the spherical head, but because it will lack smooth hyaline cartilage, the included metaphyseal region could be a contributing factor to ongoing acetabular damage and premature arthritis. These concepts help to explain why significant intraarticular damage can be seen with slips that otherwise seem to be fairly benign according to standard severity classification schemes. In contrast, impaction occurs in moderate to severe lesions where the anterolateral metaphyseal prominence is too large to enter the joint, but rather bumps against the acetabular rim and may even cause the femoral head to lever away from the acetabulum (**Fig. 4**). These abnormal mechanics can lead to not only anterosuperior labral and acetabular cartilage erosion but also posteroinferior labral separation from this

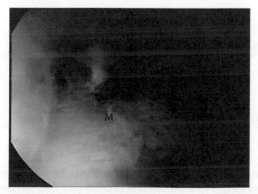

Fig. 3. Arthroscopic visualization of a ridge formed between the metaphysis (M) and epiphysis (E), which represents an inclusion type deformity.

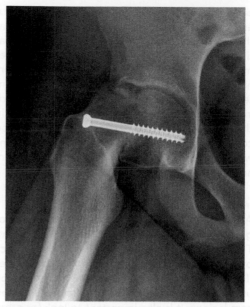

Fig. 4. .Radiograph of an impacting lesion. Contact between the metaphysis and acetabular rim is clearly evident.

contracoup lesion. An impacting deformity clinically decreases range of motion and often impairs sitting and walking ability.

Patients with SCFE also have a higher incidence of acetabular retroversion and acetabular overcoverage than their age-matched peers.[21] Both of these anatomic features in additional to the cam lesion and femoral retroversion from the slip itself contribute to a propensity for hip impingement.

ASSESSMENT
History
A patient experiencing hip impingement will classically complain of groin pain; however, many patients also note pain in the lateral thigh, buttocks, or low back. Some patients who experienced their initial SCFE symptoms in the knee may experience their subsequent impingement symptoms there as well. Symptoms tend to increase with activity, especially those requiring squatting or hip flexion, or prolonged sitting.[22] The patient may also notice decreased mobility of the hip and may have difficulties with specific activities such as riding a bicycle.

Physical Examination
Observation of the patient's gait may reveal a Trendelenburg lurch, external foot progression, or antalgic limp. With range of motion testing, the presence of obligate external rotation and abduction with hip flexion, the Drehmann sign,

can be an indicator of retroversion of the femur and FAI. Kamegaya and colleagues[23] found that the Drehmann sign was found more often in patients with less remodeling of the proximal femur and higher alpha angles. Other authors have reported hip flexion of less than 90° and internal rotation of less than 15° are reliable findings to clinically identify patients with FAI in the setting of SCFE.[19] Impingement can be confirmed with reproduction of symptoms when the hip is brought into flexion, adduction, and internal rotation.[22]

Imaging

Anteroposterior (AP) and frog-leg pelvis radiographs are often the initial images obtained. The slip angle, alpha angle, and head–neck offset can be easily measured from these images (Figs. 5 and 6). The 45° Dunn view may also be used for assessment of anterolaterally based cam lesions. It is also important to look for other abnormalities, such as acetabular retroversion, protrusion acetabuli, acetabular dysplasia, and arthritic changes. The width of the femoral neck should be very carefully assessed because severe deformities may leave the femoral neck very thin resulting in risk of femoral neck fracture during or after osteochondoroplasty (Fig. 7).

In his computer model, Rab[20] found that equivalent 2-dimensional radiographs could represent a variety of slip geometries. Therefore, 3-dimensional (3D) scans are useful for obtaining a more accurate depiction to assist with surgical planning (Fig. 8). Computed tomography (CT) scans with 3D reconstruction is preferred because it allows for better definition

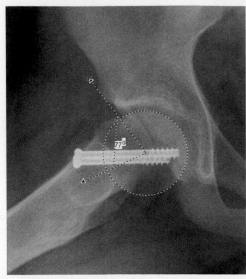

Fig. 6. Radiographic measurement of the alpha angle between a line connecting the center of the femoral head to the midpoint of the narrowest part on the femoral neck and a line from the center of the femoral head to the point where the sphericity of the femoral head ends.

of bony anatomy and can be used to generate models. MRI is less frequently used owing to difficulty with interpretation from artifact from the patient's SCFE implant, unless a second procedure is undertaken to remove it. MRI is recommended when there is concern for arthritic changes, which would be a contraindication for hip preservation procedures.

Using either CT scans or MRI, radial neck cuts allow for circumferential analysis of the head–neck junction, will better locate the cam lesion, and often reveal a larger prominence than can be appreciated on plain radiographs alone or

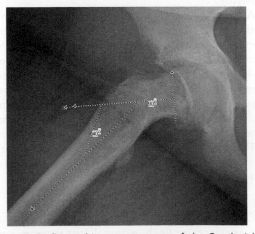

Fig. 5. Radiographic measurement of the Southwick slip angle, which is formed between a line parallel to the femoral shaft and a line perpendicular to the physis.

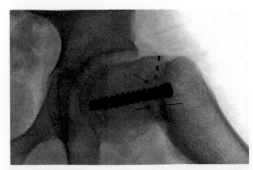

Fig. 7. Frog-leg lateral radiograph of left hip demonstrating a very thin femoral neck (*dotted line*). *Arrows* indicate the space between the femoral head and the back of the intertrochanteric portion of the proximal femur.

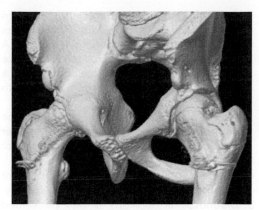

Fig. 8. Three-dimensional CT reconstruction of a post-SCFE deformity.

standard 3D imaging. The beta angle, which is formed between the femoral head–neck junction and the acetabular rim, measured on the radial view seems to correspond with cartilage damage in the superior portion of the acetabulum.[15] The average value in healthy controls is 30° versus 5° in patients with FAI.[24] The beta angle is especially useful for the assessment of SCFE deformity because it accounts for both femoral and acetabular morphology.

CT scanning is also useful for measuring femoral version. In addition to femoral retroversion being a risk factor for developing an SCFE, the deformity itself can result in epiphyseal retroversion. Severe SCFE deformity with retroversion may require open surgery including femoral derotation osteotomy.

Treatment

The management recommendations for post-SCFE deformity are centered around the degree of deformity, but also depend on the experience of the surgeon. The 3 main procedures—

arthroscopic osteochondroplasty (OCP), open OCP, and intertrochanteric osteotomy (ITO)—are described in the following sections.

Timing

When to intervene in hips with post-SCFE deformity is a controversial issue. Some patients will not report symptoms because they have consciously limited their activities and others may have little pain because of compensatory external rotation of the femur. There is reasonable evidence, however, to suggest that labral and chondral damage is occurring despite the absence of symptoms.[15] Several authors advocate for surgical correction before any symptoms develop, citing that it is easier and more effective to prevent chondral and labral damage than to treat it.[17] A few investigators have reported correction of mild deformities with hip arthroscopy at the time of in situ fixation, and observed intraarticular damage had already occurred.[25] However, no long-term studies exist to prove that early intervention alters the natural progression to arthritis.[12] Because the surgical procedures to address FAI in post-SCFE deformity are not without risk, many believe it is better to wait until a patient becomes symptomatic before offering a reconstructive surgery.

HIP ARTHROSCOPY

Similar to idiopathic FAI, the most prominent location of the cam lesion in post-SCFE deformity is the anterolateral femoral neck, making it amenable to arthroscopic OCP[26] (**Fig. 9A**).

Indications and Contraindications

The essential indication for arthroscopic OCP is a painful hip with mild deformity located along the anterolateral head–neck junction. Indications and contraindications are presented in **Table 1.**

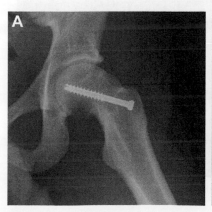
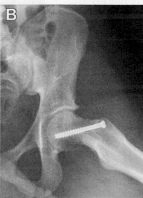

Fig. 9. (A) Preoperative radiograph of a patient with mild anterior neck prominence and (B) postoperative radiograph after arthroscopic OCP with removal of the offending prominence and normalization of head–neck offset.

Table 1
Indications and contraindications for arthroscopic OCP

Indications	Contraindications
Decreased range of motion	Severe slips
Pain with flexion and internal rotation	Cam lesion extending posterolaterally
Labral tear	Concomitant acetabular dysplasia
Articular cartilage lesions	Femoral retroversion
Mild slips	Arthritic changes with <2 mm joint space remaining
Prominence located anteriorly and laterally[26]	Patient unable to comply with restrictions or rehabilitation protocols

Surgical Technique and Procedure
Preoperative planning

- AP and frog-leg lateral pelvis radiographs are generally sufficient. The Dunn view may show a cam lesion that is located anterior-lateral.
- A CT scan can be considered for more accurate assessment of the extent and location of the deformity as well the femoral version. This imaging may confirm whether the deformity is suitable for arthroscopic management.
- MRI is indicated to rule out arthritic changes when radiographs suggest joint space narrowing, but may be difficult to interpret owing to artifact from the screw.

Preparation and patient positioning

- Supine on a traction table with either a well-padded pudendal post or using a traction pad for post-less traction. When the latter is used, the patient is placed in 10° to 15° of Trendelenburg during placement of traction. The feet are padded and placed into traction boots.

Surgical procedure

1. Fifty to 75 pounds of traction is applied, enough to distract the joint approximately 1 cm. The start time of traction should be noted, and the total time kept under 2 hours.
2. The anterolateral portal is established first, using a spinal needle and fluoroscopy to confirm intraarticular placement with a

small air arthrogram. Care must be taken not to pierce the needle through the labrum or the labrochondral junction. A flexible wire inserted through the needle should touch the medial acetabular wall. A cannula is then placed over the wire into the joint.
3. Insert a 70° arthroscope through the anterolateral portal cannula. Under direct visualization, establish a midanterior portal.
4. Create working space within the joint by performing an interportal capsulotomy.
5. Diagnostic arthroscopy is first performed within the central compartment, noting any cartilage damage (**Fig. 10**) and probing the labrum for tears.
6. If a tear in the labrum is identified, prepare the acetabular rim for anchor placement using cautery, shaver, and burr.
7. The labrum can be repaired with either vertical mattress or "luggage tag" suture configuration.
8. Small cartilage lesions can be treated with debridement and/or microfracture.
9. Release traction.
10. The cam lesion is addressed next through the peripheral compartment.
11. Extend the previously made capsulotomy over the femoral neck in a T-shaped fashion for improved visualization of the distal femoral neck.
12. Remove the SCFE screw (optional) if the physis is closed.
13. Perform dynamic arthroscopic examination to evaluate location of impingement on the labrum. Inspect the femoral head–neck junction both through the arthroscope and with fluoroscopy by flexing, abducting, and rotating the hip.

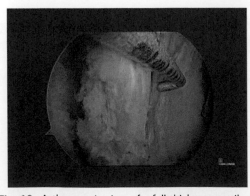

Fig. 10. Arthroscopic view of a full-thickness cartilage erosion.

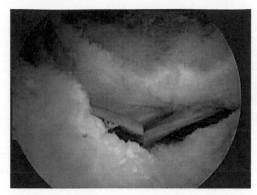

Fig. 11. Identification of the retinacular vessels for safe arthroscopic OCP.

14. Localize the retinacular vessels to determine the safe extent of OCP (**Fig. 11**).
15. Recontouring of the head–neck junction is performed with a high-speed burr. The area of maximal deformity in patients with SCFE is often at the level of the physis (**Fig. 12**). Access to the proximal extent of the cam lesion may require hip extension and/or traction. Fluoroscopy aids in identifying the abnormally prominent areas and determining when resection is adequate. Care should be taken to not remove more than 30% of the neck diameter, because biomechanical studies have shown an increased risk of neck fracture beyond this amount.[27]
16. Move the hip through a full range of motion while observing the acetabular rim for any signs of ongoing impingement and to insure a good labral seal.
17. Use fluoroscopy to confirm complete resection of cam lesion (**Fig. 9**B).
18. Close the capsule with nonabsorbable suture.

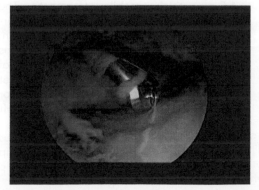

Fig. 12. Arthroscopic OCP performed at the level of the physis where maximum deformity often occurs.

Complications and their management

The overall rate of complications during hip arthroscopy is reported at 1.5% to 7.5%. Fortunately, most complications are minor with neuropraxia of the lateral femoral cutaneous nerve being the most common. Major complications are reported in less than 1% of FAI cases.[28] However, a 2017 systematic review[29] including 7 articles reporting on arthroscopy in the setting of SCFE deformity found the overall major complication rate to be slightly higher at 1.6%. This is at least partially attributed to the high proportion of patients with morbid obesity. Complications are listed in **Box 1**.

Postoperative care

The rehabilitation protocol is divided into 4 phases (**Fig. 13**). Phases II to IV typically last 4 weeks each. Return to full activities is possible by 3 months after surgery, depending on the speed of progress through each of the phases. Some patients who are poorly conditioned before surgery require longer to recover.

Outcomes

Reports from arthroscopic treatment have shown nearly ubiquitous damage to the labrum and acetabular cartilage, even when performed acutely in conjunction with in situ pinning.[25] OCP reliably improves radiographic parameters, and most patients have less pain and a better

---

Box 1
Minor and major complications of arthroscopic OCP

Minor Complications

- Neuropraxias
- 99% are transient
- Heterotopic ossification
- Iatrogenic chondral or labral injury
- Superficial wound infection

Major Complications

- Deep infection
- Pulmonary emboli

Abdominal compartment syndrome from extravasation of fluid into abdomen

- Avascular necrosis of the femoral head
- Vascular injury
- Femoral neck fracture
- Dislocation

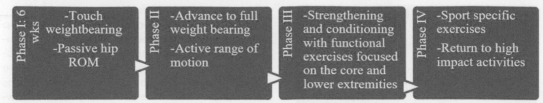

Fig. 13. Rehabilitation phases after hip arthroscopy with OCP. ROM, range of motion.

range of motion at short-term follow-up (Table 2).

OPEN OSTEOCHONDROPLASTY

When the deformity is too large or complex for arthroscopic treatment, surgical hip dislocation (SHD) allows 360° access to the femoral head and neck for open OCP as well as evaluation and treatment of intraarticular pathology.[19] Because the amount of bone that can be resected from the femoral neck is limited, open OCP may be combined with a flexion/rotation ITO for further correction as well as to address concomitant alterations in the neck shaft axis and femoral retroversion.

Indications and Contraindications

The primary indication for open OCP is a moderate to severe slip where the metaphyseal ridge extends beyond the anterosuperior surface of the neck (Fig. 14A). Table 3 provides the other major indications as well as contraindications. Open treatment is also preferred over arthroscopy when other aspects of femoral deformity, such as femoral retroversion or coxa vara, will also be treated.

Surgical Technique and Procedure
Preoperative planning

- AP, frog-leg, and Dunn view pelvis radiographs are obtained.
- CT scan of the pelvis and femur with radial neck cuts and 3D reconstruction allows for complete analysis of the deformity, including femoral version.

Preparation and patient positioning

- The patient is placed in a lateral decubitus position and stabilized on a peg board with posts on a radiolucent table. Beanbags may be used, but are more likely to impede free rotation of the leg.
  ○ Bony prominences on the down side should be well-padded.

- A pillow is placed between the legs to maintain the hip in abduction and the operative leg parallel to the floor.

Surgical approach

- Surgical hip dislocation as described by Ganz and associates is undertaken.[32]

Surgical procedure

1. Make an approximately 12-cm longitudinal incision centered over the greater trochanter. The incision will need to extend further distally if an ITO is planned.
2. Split the iliotibial band in line with its fibers and the incision. Proximally, carry the split between the gluteus maximus posteriorly and tensor fascia lata anteriorly (Gibson interval).
3. Internally rotate the hip to obtain access to the posterior aspect of the greater trochanter and short external rotators. Identify the piriformis tendon and so that the underlying vasculature can be protected. Identify the interval between the piriformis and gluteus minimus.
4. Distally, incise the fascia of the vastus lateralis near its posterior border. Staying extraperiosteal, elevate the muscle anteriorly.
5. Perform an osteotomy of the greater trochanter, aiming for an approximately 1.5-cm thick mobile fragment. The trigastric osteotomy should begin anterior-lateral to the piriformis tendon insertion, exit just deep to the gluteus medius proximally, and contain the entire origin of the vastus lateralis. A saw blade that oscillates only at the tip is useful for gaining leverage against posterior soft tissue. Mobilize the fragment anteriorly.
6. Gently elevate the fibers of the gluteus minimus to expose the underlying hip capsule. Flex and externally rotate the hip to assist in anterior exposure.
7. Make a Z-shaped capsulotomy. The transverse limb is made first and begins at

Table 2
Reported outcomes following arthroscopic OCP for post-SCFE deformity

Study	No. of Hips	Follow-up (mo), Mean (Range)	Findings	Outcomes
Basheer et al,[26] 2016	18	29 (23–56)	12 had labral damage; Only 2 were amenable to repair 4 had Outerbridge grade 3–4 cartilage damage and underwent microfracture	Alpha angle improved from 91.6° to 51.7° Flexion improved from 76 to 110 IR improved from 0 to 9 All had pain relief; 56% had complete relief Mean mHHS improved from 56.2 to 75.1 Mean NAHS scores improved from 52.1 to 73.6 Longer time to surgery associated with worse outcomes
Chen et al,[30] 2014	34	22 (12–56)	All had labral damage 26 hips had acetabular cartilage abrasion	Alpha angle significantly improved from 88° to 55° IR in flexion improved from −21 to +10 88% achieved complete pain relief 2 patients had mild residual pain 2 patients with residual obligate ER in flexion underwent correction with subsequent open osteotomies
Lee et al,[10] 2013	5	(3–36)	Synovitis, labral injury, and/or cartilage damage anterosuperiorly	Alpha angle improved from a mean of 76.8° to 43° All pain free with improved range of motion
Leunig et al,[25] 2010	3	(3–23)	Labral fraying, acetabular chondromalacia, and a prominent metaphyseal ridge	Alpha angle was improved by 34°–40° Head–neck offset was improved by 4.5–5.9 mm All had improvement in flexion and IR All were pain free in unrestricted activity
Tscholl et al,[31] 2016	14	Not reported	3 had labral fraying 2 had Beck grade I cartilage damage 2 had Beck grade III cartilage damage	Mean alpha angle improved from 57° to 37°

Abbreviations: ER, external rotation; IR, internal rotation; mHHS, modified Harris Hip Score; NAHS, nonarthritic hip score.

A **B**

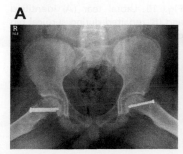 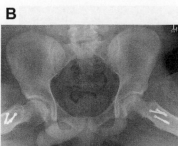

Fig. 14. (A) Radiographs of a patient with bilateral slips who was treated with (B) open OCP via surgical hip dislocation.

Table 3
Indications and contraindications for open OCP

Indications	Contraindications
Moderate to severe slips	Anterior hip instability
Metaphyseal prominence extending posterolaterally	Advanced arthritic changes
Coxa breva or high riding trochanter	Patient unable to comply with restrictions or rehabilitation protocols
Labral tears requiring reconstruction	
Coxa profunda or global overcoverage, which make arthroscopy more difficult	

the anterosuperior corner of the stable trochanter traveling anterolaterally along the axis of the femoral neck. The second limb is made inferiorly on the neck traveling anteriorly toward the lesser trochanter but should remain anterior to it. The final limb is a sharp posterior turn from the first along the acetabular rim to the level of the piriformis. The labrum should be identified and protected.

8. Subluxate the hip anteriorly and release the ligamentum teres with a curved scissor and excise the remnant from the acetabulum and the fovea.
9. Range the hip and note areas of impingement.
10. Dislocate the femoral head using a bone hook under the neck for gentle traction while flexing and externally rotating the leg. The foot is placed into a sterile pouch anteriorly. The retinaculum containing the terminal medial femoral circumflex artery branches should be identified and protected on the posterosuperior aspect of the neck.
11. Epiphyseal perfusion is confirmed with the head in a dislocated position. Drill one or two 2.0 holes into the head for direct observation of bleeding or for introduction of a sterile intracranial pressure probe or arterial line.
12. Expose the acetabulum for assessment and treatment of any intraarticular damage (**Fig. 15**).
13. OCP of the femoral head and neck is then performed using a combination of curved osteotome, rongeur, and high-speed 5-mm burr. Hemispherical guides may be used to confirm sphericity of the anterior head–neck junction. The hip should be reduced periodically and put through a full range of motion for evaluation of the head–neck contour and any areas of impingement. Fluoroscopy should be used frequently to ensure the femoral neck is not becoming too thin.
14. Vascularity is assessed again through the previously made drill holes. Bleeding cancellous bone in the area of the OCP made proximal to the physis is additional evidence of adequate perfusion.
15. Reapproximate the capsule. Avoid excessive tightening because this can create too much tension on the retinacular vessels.
16. Advance the mobile trochanter distally until the tip is level with the center of the femoral head and secure with three 3.5- to 4.5-mm screws in a triangular pattern (**Fig. 14**B).
17. If concomitant femoral ITO is planned, it is performed at this point. The trochanter can be fixed as described elsewhere in this article, and the femoral plate placed below the trochanter. Alternatively, the plate can be placed over the trochanter and be used to fixate both the trochanter and the ITO.

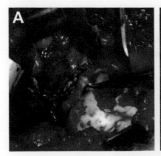
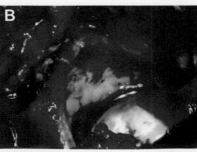

Fig. 15. Labral tear (A) identified and (B) repaired during surgical hip dislocation.

Complications and their management

Surgical hip dislocation is a safe procedure when performed by experienced surgeons.[33] Avascular necrosis is the most feared complication, but a clear understanding and protection of the retinacular vessels minimizes this risk. The overall rate of major complications is higher than arthroscopy at 10.7%. Trochanteric nonunion is the most frequent event and reason for revision surgery.[29] Major and minor complications are presented in Box 2.

Postoperative care

The first several weeks after surgery are focused on protecting capsular closure and trochanteric fixation while maintaining range of motion. Passive range of motion is initiated immediately with a continuous passive motion machine to minimize the risk for hip adhesions. Anterior hip dislocation precautions are recommended, and hip adduction and external rotation are avoided. Active abduction is avoided for the first 6 weeks to protect trochanteric fixation. After a 6-week healing period, gait training, strengthening, and return to activities are permitted in a graduated fashion. Return to high impact sports occurs around 6 months postoperatively and should be supervised by a physical therapist (Fig. 16).

Outcomes

Few authors have reported on isolated OCP for post-SCFE deformity, and there are no long-term studies assessing patient-reported outcome measures or arthritis progression. Short-term outcomes show improvement in both objective radiographic parameters and range of motion, as well as patient reported pain and function (Table 4).

INTERTROCHANTERIC OSTEOTOMY

As described in the previous section, ITO can be used in isolation or as a combined procedure with open OCP via surgical hip dislocation or a limited anterior approach.[37]

Indications and Contraindications

ITO is a powerful correction tool to address impingement, malrotation, and coxa vara (Fig. 17A). The ability to correct femoral retroversion is an important element because it contributes to obligate external rotation, which can be functionally limiting, and external foot progression, which can adversely affect knee kinematics and be cosmetically displeasing.[38] In a study assessing outcomes from arthroscopic management of primary FAI, Fabricant and colleagues[39] found that patients with less than 5° of anteversion improved much less than those with normal or increased version, but this relationship has not been well studied in post-SCFE deformity. A list of indications and contraindications is provided in Table 5.

Surgical Technique and Procedure
Preoperative planning

- AP and frog-leg lateral radiographs are obtained.
  - Measure the epiphyseal–diaphyseal angle on the frog-leg view to determine the required amount of flexion to bring the shaft in line with the neck. If the intended angular correction is greater than 35°, a resulting z-deformity of the proximal femur may complicate future arthroplasty stem insertion.[40] To minimize this risk, use caution intraoperatively to keep the shaft aligned with the piriformis fossa.
  - Measure the neck-shaft angle to determine whether the correction should also be valgus producing. If the contralateral hip is normal, it is used as a template.
- A magnetic resonance arthrogram may be necessary to evaluate for labral tears, cartilage damage, and avascular necrosis, any of which would alter the treatment plan.
- A CT scan with 3D reconstruction is useful for determining whether an isolated or combined procedure is indicated.

Box 2
Complications after open OCP

Minor Complications
- Heterotopic ossification
- Superficial wound infection

Major Complications
- Trochanteric nonunion
- Iatrogenic cartilage and/or labral damage
- Avascular necrosis
- Femoral neck fracture
- Instability
- Nerve injury
- Deep vein thrombosis
- Deep infection

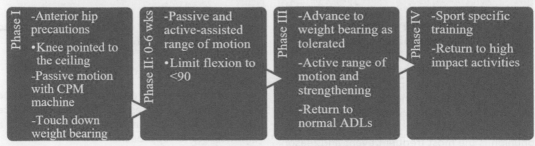

Phase I
-Anterior hip precautions
• Knee pointed to the ceiling
-Passive motion with CPM machine
-Touch down weight bearing

Phase II: 0-6 wks
-Passive and active-assisted range of motion
• Limit flexion to <90

Phase III
-Advance to weight bearing as tolerated
-Active range of motion and strengthening
-Return to normal ADLs

Phase IV
-Sport specific training
-Return to high impact activities

Fig. 16. Phases of rehabilitation after open OCP. ADLs, activities of daily living. CPM, continuous passive motion machine.

- A CT scan or MRI rotational profile is obtained (optional).

Preparation and patient positioning

- The patient is placed in lateral decubitus or supine on a radiolucent table.

Surgical approach

- A lateral approach to the proximal femur is taken.

Surgical procedure

1. Make an approximately 12-cm incision from the tip of the greater trochanter extending distally in line with the femoral shaft.
2. Incise the iliotibial band longitudinally. The fibers of the vastus lateralis fascia are visible beneath the split. Incise the fascia off the vastus lateralis longitudinally near its

posterior border from the distal portion of the incision up to the level of the vastus ridge. Create a T in the fascia just distal to the vastus ridge and extend this anteriorly while protecting the fibers of the gluteus medius. Elevate the vastus subperiosteally in an anterior direction.

3. Insert a guidewire centrally in the femoral neck as seen on the lateral view. Insert a Steinmann pin through the femoral condyles, perpendicular to the tibia. The angle made by these pins approximates the femoral version (**Fig. 18**). Place the initial guide pins for a proximal femoral locking plate or a blade plate chisel oriented anteriorly to match the planned angle of flexion.
4. Plan the level of the osteotomy at or slightly above the lesser trochanter according to the specific implant guide. Dissect

Table 4 Outcomes after open OCP			
Study	**Patients**	**Follow-up Period**	**Outcomes**
Erickson et al,[34] 2017	13[a]	61.7 (23–120)	Mean slip angle improved 40.7° Mean alpha angle of 55.8° at final follow-up No cases of avascular necrosis 1 osteotomy nonunion
Rebello et al,[35] 2009	7 OCP 8 OCP + ITO	Not reported	Improved WOMAC scores for pain, stiffness, and function
Spencer et al,[36] 2006	6 OCP 6 OCP + ITO	16 (8–25) 12 10–14)	For OCP + ITO, 5/6 had improved WOMAC and function scores and flexion/IR improved from −20 to +10 For OCP, 4/6 had improved WOMAC and function scores Patients with chondral flaps tended to have less pain relief and worse function SCFE patients had better outcomes than a comparative group of idiopathic FAI

Abbreviations: IR, internal rotation; WOMAC, Western Ontario and McMaster Universities Osteoarthritis Index.
[a] Subset treated greater than 6 mo from time of in situ pinning.

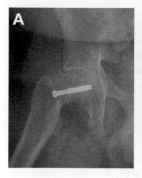
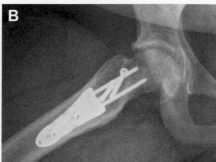

Fig. 17. Radiographs of patient with (A) a severe slip who was treated with (B) combined open OCP and ITO.

circumferentially around the femur at this site, and place Hohman retractors for protection of the soft tissues.
5. Make the first osteotomy cut perpendicular to the shaft. The second osteotomy is started from the same location on the lateral cortex of the proximal fragment and angled proximally to create the anteriorly based wedge according to the clinical appearance of the deformity and preoperative templating.
6. Attach the implant to the proximal fragment. Choose an implant with the neck-shaft angle that most closely approximates the desired amount of valgus.
7. Reduce the shaft to the plate with a clamp, then internally rotate the leg to correct retroversion. The previously placed guide pins can be "dialed" down to the desired angle of anteversion. Hip rotation should be compared with the contralateral side, if it is normal. Secure the implant using at least one compression screw adjacent to the osteotomy and 2 to 3 additional screws distally (Fig. 17B).

Complications and their management
Several possible adverse outcomes are possible after ITO (Box 3), but most authors report only a few cases with complications after ITO for post-SCFE deformity (Table 6).

Table 5
Indications and contraindications for ITO

Indications	Contraindications
Moderate to severe slips	Intraarticular pathology (indication for combined SHD)
Inability to obtain 90° hip flexion or at least neutral internal rotation with OCP alone	Metaphyseal corner impingement (indication for combined SHD)
Symptomatic femoral retroversion	Advanced degenerative changes
Obligate external rotation impeding activities of daily living	Patient unable to comply with restrictions or rehabilitation protocols
Knee pain from external foot progression	Acute SCFE (controversial)[40]
Coxa vara	
Focal avascular necrosis of the femoral head that can be moved out of the weight bearing portion with the osteotomy correction	

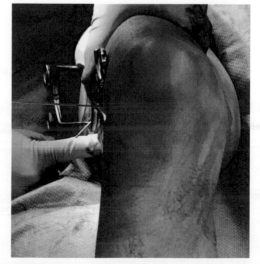

Fig. 18. Intraoperative assessment of femoral version using a Steinmann pin placed perpendicular to the tibia referenced to a guide pin in the center of the femoral neck. Version in this case is approximately 45°.

Box 3
Minor and major complications of ITO
Minor Complications
• Neuropraxia
• Delayed union
• Prominent implant
• Superficial wound infection
Major Complications
• Nonunion
• Malrotation
• Avascular necrosis
• Chondrolysis
• Implant failure
• Deep infection
• Deep vein thrombosis

Postoperative care

The initial phase of recovery after ITO limits activity while the osteotomy site heals. Progressive motion and strengthening are initiated in a similar fashion as described for OCP once satisfactory healing has occurred (**Fig. 19**).

Outcomes

ITO has been performed for SCFE deformity for more than 60 years with demonstrated effectiveness and safety.[41] As seen in **Table 6**, the majority of patients have good to excellent clinical and radiological outcomes. The improved understanding that articular damage begins accumulating shortly after an SCFE suggests that earlier intervention could potentially lead to better results in the future.

Table 6
Reported outcomes following ITO

Study	Patients/Hips	Follow-up (y)	Outcomes
Kartenbender et al,[42] 2000	35/39	23.4 (19–27)	77% had good to excellent Southwick scores 67% were radiographically good to excellent[a] 46% walked with a moderate to severe limp 3 developed advanced arthritis 2 developed avascular necrosis
Saisu et al,[43] 2013	32/32	5 (2–9)	94% were without pain or daily inconvenience 75% had a negative impingement sign 8 patients had persistent Drehman's sign Beta angles decreased by mean 39° Alpha angles did not change significantly 75% were Kellgren-Lewis grade 1 3% developed chondrolysis No cases of postoperative avascular necrosis
Trisolino et al,[41] 2017	39/47	18.9 (1–39)	68.5% survivorship free from total hip replacement at 39 y 2 developed avascular necrosis, 2 developed chondrolysis Mean HOOS 82.4% 16/22 had Tonnis grade 0 or I arthritic changes Older age at surgery and avascular necrosis or chondrolysis negatively affected prognosis
Witbreuk et al,[44] 2009	28/32	8.2 (2.0–25.7)	71% had excellent or good HHS SF-36 equivalent to age matched population 80% were Kellgren-Lewis grade 0 or 1 Flexion and internal rotation improved by mean 11° and 37° respectively

Abbreviations: HOOS, hip orthopedic outcome score; HHS, Harris hip score; SF-36, short form-36; SHD, surgical hip dislocation.
[a] Southwick classification.

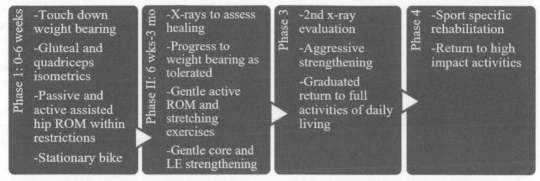

Fig. 19. Phases of rehabilitation after ITO. LE, lower extremity; ROM, range of motion.

SUMMARY

The techniques described for treating post-SCFE deformity have demonstrated effectiveness for reducing symptoms related to FAI and correcting the radiographic and clinical signs that are associated with progressive degenerative changes. However, the application of arthroscopic and open OCP for SCFE is an evolving field with only short-term results available. The data for ITO span a longer time period, but still only capture patients who are in their 20s or 30s. For symptomatic patients, the decision to intervene is fairly straightforward with a goal of improving symptoms. How to intervene depends on the nature of the deformity and the experience of the surgeon with the different surgical techniques. Difficulty arises when considering whether asymptomatic patients with decreased range of motion, obligate external rotation, femoral retroversion, and/or radiographic evidence of FAI pathology should be treated prophylactically. Several authors argue that the intervention is likely to be more successful if performed before irreversible damage occurs.[17] The theoretic arguments are compelling, but we do not yet have evidence to show that treating post-SCFE deformity will change the natural progression toward early arthritis.[12] Given the real, albeit small, potential for complications, the judgment of whom to operate on and when is an imperative avenue of future research.

REFERENCES

1. Novais EN, Millis MB. Slipped capital femoral epiphysis: prevalence, pathogenesis, and natural history. Clin Orthop Relat Res 2012;470(12):3432–8.
2. Mullins MM, Sood M, Hashemi-Nejad A, et al. The management of avascular necrosis after slipped capital femoral epiphysis. J Bone Joint Surg Br 2005;87-B:1669–74.
3. Sankar WN, Vanderhave KL, Matheney T, et al. The modified Dunn procedure for unstable slipped capital femoral epiphysis: a multicenter perspective. J Bone Joint Surg Am 2013;95(7):585–91.
4. Kuzyk PR, Kim YJ, Millis MB. Surgical management of healed slipped capital femoral epiphysis. J Am Acad Orthop Surg 2011;19:667–77.
5. Castañeda P, Macías C, Rocha A, et al. Functional outcome of stable grade III slipped capital femoral epiphysis treated with in situ pinning. J Pediatr Orthop 2009;29:454–8.
6. Larson AN, Sierra RJ, Yu EM, et al. Outcomes of slipped capital femoral epiphysis treated with in situ pinning. J Pediatr Orthop 2012;32(2):125–30.
7. Ganz RP, Parvizi J, Beck M, et al. Femoroacetabular impingement: a cause for osteoarthritis of the hip. Clin Orthop Relat Res 2003;417:112–20.
8. Castañeda P, Ponce C, Villareal G, et al. The natural history of osteoarthritis after a slipped capital femoral epiphysis/the pistol grip deformity. J Pediatr Orthop 2013;33:S76–82.
9. Hosalkar HS, Pandya NK, Bomar JD, et al. Hip impingement in slipped capital femoral epiphysis: a changing perspective. J Child Orthop 2012;6(3):161–72.
10. Lee CB, Matheney T, Yen YM. Case reports: acetabular damage after mild slipped capital femoral epiphysis. Clin Orthop Relat Res 2013;471(7):2163–72.
11. Ziebarth K, Leunig M, Slongo T, et al. Slipped capital femoral epiphysis: relevant pathophysiological findings with open surgery. Clin Orthop Relat Res 2013;471(7):2156–62.
12. Wiemann JM, Herrera-Soto JA. Can we alter the natural history of osteoarthritis after SCFE with early realignment? J Pediatr Orthop 2013;33:S83–7.
13. Wensaas A, Gunderson RB, Svenningsen S, et al. Femoroacetabular impingement after slipped upper femoral epiphysis: the radiological diagnosis and clinical outcome at long-term follow-up. J Bone Joint Surg Br 2012;94-B:1487–93.

14. Dawes BJ, Jaremko JL, Balakumar J. Radiographic assessment of bone remodelling in slipped upper femoral epiphyses using Klein's line and the a angle of femoral- acetabular impingement: a retrospective review. J Pediatr Orthop 2011;31:153–8.

15. Zilkens C, Miese F, Krauspe R, et al. Symptomatic femoroacetabular impingement: does the offset decrease correlate with cartilage damage? A pilot study. Clin Orthop Relat Res 2013;471(7):2173–82.

16. Fraitzl CR, Käfer W, Nelitz M, et al. Radiological evidence of femoroacetabular impingement in mild slipped capital femoral epiphysis: a mean follow-up of 14.4 years after pinning in situ. J Bone Joint Surg Br 2007;89-B:1592–6.

17. Millis MB, Novais EN. In situ fixation for slipped capital femoral epiphysis: perspectives in 2011. J Bone Joint Surg Am 2011;93(Suppl 2):46–51.

18. Souder CD, Bomar JD, Wenger DR. The role of capital realignment versus in situ stabilization for the treatment of slipped capital femoral epiphysis. J Pediatr Orthop 2014;34:791–8.

19. Mahran MA, Baraka MM, Hefny HM. Slipped capital femoral epiphysis: a review of management in the hip impingement era. SICOT J 2017;3:35.

20. Rab G. The geometry of slipped capital femoral epiphysis: implications for movement, impingement, and corrective osteotomy. J Pediatr Orthop 1999;19:419–24.

21. Sankar WN, Brighton BK, Kim YJ, et al. Acetabular morphology in slipped capital femoral epiphysis. J Pediatr Orthop 2011;31:254–8.

22. Clohisy JC, Knaus ER, Hunt DM, et al. Clinical presentation of patients with symptomatic anterior hip impingement. Clin Orthop Relat Res 2009;467(3):638–44.

23. Kamegaya M, Saisu T, Nakamura J, et al. Drehmann sign and femoro-acetabular impingement in SCFE. J Pediatr Orthop 2011;31:853–7.

24. Wyss TF, Clark JM, Weishaupt D, et al. Correlation between internal rotation and bony anatomy in the hip. Clin Orthop Relat Res 2007;460:152–8.

25. Leunig M, Horowitz K, Manner H, et al. In situ pinning with arthroscopic osteoplasty for mild SCFE: a preliminary technical report. Clin Orthop Relat Res 2010;468(12):3160–7.

26. Basheer SZ, Cooper AP, Maheshwari R, et al. Arthroscopic treatment of femoroacetabular impingement following slipped capital femoral epiphysis. Bone Joint J 2016;98-B:21–7.

27. Mardones RM, Gonzalez C, Chen Q, et al. Surgical treatment of femoroacetabular impingement: evaluation of the effect of the size of the resection. J Bone Joint Surg Am 2005;87-A(2):273–9.

28. Kuhns BD, Frank RM, Pulido L. Open and arthroscopic surgical treatment of femoroacetabular impingement. Front Surg 2015;2:63.

29. Oduwole KO, de Sa D, Kay J, et al. Surgical treatment of femoroacetabular impingement following slipped capital femoral epiphysis: a systematic review. Bone Joint Res 2017;6(8):472–80.

30. Chen A, Youderian A, Watkins S, et al. Arthroscopic femoral neck osteoplasty in slipped capital femoral epiphysis. Arthroscopy 2014;30(10):1229–34.

31. Tscholl PM, Zingg PO, Dora C, et al. Arthroscopic osteochondroplasty in patients with mild slipped capital femoral epiphysis after in situ fixation. J Child Orthop 2016;10(1):25–30.

32. Ganz R, Gill TJ, Gautier E, et al. Surgical dislocation of the adult hip: a technique with full access to the femoral head and acetabulum without the risk of avascular necrosis. J Bone Joint Surg Br 2001;83-B:1119–24.

33. McClincy MP, Bosch PP. Combined surgical dislocation and proximal femoral osteotomy for correction of SCFE-induced femoroacetabular impingement. Oper Tech Orthop 2013;23(3):140–5.

34. Erickson JB, Samora WP, Klingele KE. Treatment of chronic, stable slipped capital femoral epiphysis via surgical hip dislocation with combined osteochondroplasty and Imhauser osteotomy. J Child Orthop 2017;11(4):284–8.

35. Rebello G, Spencer S, Millis MB, et al. Surgical dislocation in the management of pediatric and adolescent hip deformity. Clin Orthop Relat Res 2009;467(3):724–31.

36. Spencer S, Millis B, Kim YJ. Early results of treatment for hip impingement syndrome in slipped capital femoral epiphysis and pistol grip deformity of the femoral head-neck junction using the surgical dislocation technique. J Pediatr Orthop 2006;26:281–5.

37. Azegami S, Kosuge D, Ramachandran M. Surgical treatment of femoroacetabular impingement in patients with slipped capital femoral epiphysis: a review of current surgical techniques. Bone Joint J 2013;95-B:445–51.

38. Stevens PM, Anderson L, MacWilliams BA. Femoral shaft osteotomy for obligate outward rotation due to SCFE. Strategies Trauma Limb Reconstr 2017;12(1):27–33.

39. Fabricant PD, Fields KG, Taylor SA, et al. The effect of femoral and acetabular version on clinical outcomes after arthroscopic femoroacetabular impingement surgery. J Bone Joint Surg Am 2015;97(7):537–43.

40. Schai PA, Exner GU. Corrective Imhauser intertrochanteric osteotomy. Oper Orthop Traumatol 2007;19(4):368–88.

41. Trisolino G, Pagliazzi G, Di Gennaro GL, et al. Long-term results of combined epiphysiodesis and Imhauser intertrochanteric osteotomy in SCFE: a retrospective study on 53 hips. J Pediatr Orthop 2017;37(6):409–15.

42. Kartenbender K, Cordier W, Katthagen BD. Long-term follow-up study after corrective Imhauser osteotomy for severe slipped capital femoral epiphysis. J Pediatr Orthop 2000;20:749–56.

43. Saisu T, Kamegaya M, Segawa Y, et al. Postoperative improvement of femoroacetabular impingement after intertrochanteric flexion osteotomy for SCFE. Clin Orthop Relat Res 2013;471(7): 2183–91.

44. Witbreuk MM, Bolkenbaas M, Mullender MG, et al. The results of downgrading moderate and severe slipped capital femoral epiphysis by an early Imhauser femur osteotomy. J Child Orthop 2009; 3(5):405–10.

Pediatric Anterior Cruciate Ligament Reconstruction

Crystal A. Perkins, MD*, S. Clifton Willimon, MD

KEYWORDS

- Anterior cruciate ligament • ACL Reconstruction • Pediatric • Adolescent • Knee
- Skeletally immature

KEY POINTS

- Anterior cruciate ligament injuries are the most common cause of traumatic knee effusion in adolescents and are occurring with an increasing incidence.
- Assessment of skeletal age and growth remaining is critical to treating skeletally immature patients with anterior cruciate ligament tears.
- Nonoperative treatment of anterior cruciate ligament tears, even in the youngest patient, is associated with secondary chondral and meniscal injury and is not appropriate for the majority of patients.
- Physeal-sparing, partial transphyseal, and transphyseal anterior cruciate ligament reconstructions allow for stabilization of the knee while respecting the various amounts of growth remaining of children and adolescents.

INTRODUCTION

Anterior cruciate ligament (ACL) injuries in children and adolescents have increased in prevalence in the last 2 decades. According to recent estimates, ACL injuries in this population occur with an incidence of 14 per 100,000 exposures.[1] ACL reconstructions in patients younger than 15 years increased by 425% from 1994 to 2006.[2] An increasing number of young athletes (38 million participating in organized sports in 2009 to 2010),[1] year-round sports participation, and earlier single sport specialization have all been proposed as theories for this trend.[3,4]

Historically, skeletally immature athletes with ACL tears were managed with activity modification and bracing, largely owing to concern for physeal damage from standard reconstruction techniques. However, there are significant risks of secondary chondral and meniscal damage associated with delayed reconstruction.[5,6] As the evidence in support of early reconstruction has accumulated, practice patterns have changed in favor of operative intervention. An

understanding of physeal anatomy and reconstructive options is vital when planning surgery for children and adolescents with ACL injuries. The purpose of this article is to review the anatomy of the ACL and pediatric knee, imaging and diagnosis of ACL injuries, and unique operative techniques for treatment of these injuries in skeletally immature children and adolescents.

ANATOMY AND FUNCTION OF THE ANTERIOR CRUCIATE LIGAMENT

The ACL is the primary restraint of anterior translation and rotation of the tibia on the femur and is maximally loaded at 30° of flexion.[7] The ACL originates on the lateral femoral condyle and inserts on the medial intercondylar spine of the tibia. As the knee passes through a range of motion, the ligament changes in orientation, from more vertical in extension and horizontal in flexion.[8] The lateral bifurcate ridge separates the anteromedial bundle and posterolateral bundles of the ACL within the femoral footprint, but the bundles are named

---

Disclosure Statement: The authors have nothing to disclose.
Children's Healthcare of Atlanta, 5445 Meridian Mark Road, Suite 250, Atlanta, GA 30342, USA
* Corresponding author.
E-mail address: crystal.perkins@choa.org

based on their insertion on the tibia.[9] The ACL is not an isometric structure. As the bundles change in orientation through a range of motion, the anteromedial bundle is tight at high-flexion angles and the posterolateral bundle is tight at low-flexion angles.[10]

The origin and insertion of the ACL are in close proximity to the distal femoral and proximal tibial physes. Authors have described the relationship of the origin and insertions of the ACL to the distal femoral and proximal tibial physis.[11–13] An understanding of physeal anatomy is vital when planning surgery for children and adolescents with ACL injuries and open physes.

CLINICAL EVALUATION OF AN ANTERIOR CRUCIATE LIGAMENT TEAR

A high index of suspicion for an intra-articular injury must be had for all patients with a traumatic knee injury and an effusion. ACL tears are the most common cause of an acute traumatic knee hemarthrosis.[14] Patients with a knee effusion who report a pop in the knee after an acute knee injury have a 70% chance of an ACL tear.[14] ACL tears and patellar dislocations or subluxations are easily confused. An effusion, lateral knee pain and tenderness, and injury sustained from a jump landing or while pivoting are common findings in ACL injury patients, but also patients with a patellar subluxation or dislocation. We frequently diagnose patients with an ACL tear after a reported history or even treatment for presumed patellofemoral instability. Careful examination is necessary to avoid this diagnostic pitfall.

The physical examination of the knee is critical to diagnosis of ACL injuries, as well as concomitant injuries such as collateral ligament or meniscal tears. Dynamic examinations, such as the Lachman and pivot shift, should be compared with the uninjured knee. In these young patients, examination of the uninjured knee is essential to allow assessment of physiologic laxity, which is often present in this age group. Additionally, an examination of the well leg allows the patient to experience the examination maneuvers performed on the uninjured, and nonpainful, limb helping to relax the patient in this often-anxious age group. Initial imaging should include AP, lateral, notch, and sunrise views of the injured knee to assess for physeal status, fractures, and other underlying problems such as osteochondritis dissecans. In skeletally immature patients, standing long-leg alignment radiographs are important to assess for limb length inequalities or angular deformities. A posteroanterior left hand radiograph is also necessary in skeletally immature patients to determine skeletal age and is the authors' favored method for calculating skeletal age and growth remaining. MRI is the gold standard imaging modality for the diagnosis of ligament, meniscus, and chondral injuries of the knee. Recognition of associated injuries is critical to surgical planning and optimal treatment of traumatic knee injuries.

ASSESSING SKELETAL MATURITY

The physes about the knee produce substantial growth of the lower extremity with the distal femoral physis contributing 70% of femoral growth (9 mm/y) and the proximal tibial physis contributing 60% of tibial growth (6 mm/y). Assessments of skeletal maturity in the literature have historically been done by chronologic age, presence of an open physis on plain radiography, Tanner staging of secondary sexual characteristics, bone age, and combinations of these methods. Chronologic age and the presence of an open physis on radiographs are notoriously inaccurate. Tanner staging is based on dividing secondary sexual characteristics into 1 of 5 groups.[15] These stages parallel the adolescent growth spurt and subsequent closure of the physes. Unfortunately, they do not seem to be accurate; a study of experienced physicians performing these assessments has shown them not to be reliable or reproducible.[16,17] Additionally, Tanner staging has not been documented to predict the growth remaining at the distal femoral and proximal tibial physes.

Bone age uses a posterior-anterior radiograph of the left hand, which is then compared with standard examples in the Greulich-Pyle atlas.[18] Although perhaps one of the more objective methods available to us, there is a great deal of overlap and indetermination for any given radiograph. A shorthand version is now available but still relies on the standards from the Gruelich-Pyle dataset and assessment.[19]

In an attempt to determine the age at which it is feasible to perform a transphyseal ACL reconstruction, multiple authors have categorized patients into treatment groups based on Tanner stage and predictions of growth remaining. One such algorithm groups patients as prepubescent (Tanner stage 1–2, bone age <12 years in males and <11 years in females), pubescent (Tanner stage 3–4, bone age 13–16 years in males and 12–14 years in females), or older adolescents (Tanner stage 5, bone age >16 years in males and >14 years in females).[20] Based on bone age, treatment recommendations are that prepubescent patients are treated with physeal-sparing reconstructions, adolescent patients with transphyseal reconstruction with soft tissue grafts, and older adolescents with a conventional ACL reconstruction with either soft tissue or bone–patellar tendon–bone grafts.[20]

Guzzanti and associates[21] introduced the concept of growth remaining and proposed categorizing children into 3 groups based on their risk for growth disturbance (high, intermediate, and low). High risk were preadolescents who had a lower extremity growth potential of more than 7 cm and included Tanner stage 1 children with a bone age in females of less than 11 years and in males of less than 12 years. The intermediate group had lower extremity growth potential of 5 to 7 cm and included Tanner stages 2 and 3 and bone age in females 11 to 13 years and in males 12 to 15 years. Last, the low-risk patients had less than 5 cm of growth remaining and included Tanner stages 4 and 5 and bone age in females greater than 14 years and males greater than 16 years. Using this algorithm, partial transphyseal reconstructions in 10 patients deemed at intermediate risk and followed to skeletal maturity (24–108 months) resulted in no significant limb length discrepancies.[21]

Kelly and Dimeglio[22] have published tables that illustrate the growth remaining of the distal femur and proximal tibia based on a patient's bone age (Fig. 1). These tables effectively group patients in to 3 groups based on combined growth remaining around the knee: less than 1 cm, 1 to 5 cm, and more than 5 cm. The authors use Dimeglio's principal of growth remaining to guide their ACL reconstruction technique, and this is described further in the Preferred Approach section.

The goal of ACL reconstruction is to restore knee stability while protecting growth. The risk of physeal damage with limb length discrepancy and angular deformity has to be weighed against the risk of leaving the knee unstable in these highly active youth who have a limited propensity to self-restrict from risky activities. Physicians taking care of ACL tears in skeletally immature patients should be proficient in assessing growth remaining, understanding and minimizing the risks of traditional transphyseal ACL reconstruction based on basic science and clinical evidence, choosing between a transphyseal technique or other alternatives such as physeal-sparing reconstructions, and monitoring patients after surgery for potential growth disturbances.

PHYSEAL ANATOMY AND ANTERIOR CRUCIATE LIGAMENT RECONSTRUCTION

Numerous animal studies have helped to define the anatomy of the physis and its response to trauma. As early as 1959, Campbell and co-workers[23] described growth retardation that resulted from a single large hole drilled through the open physes of dogs and complete growth arrest from cortical bone placed across a transphyseal tunnel. Tunnel size can also impact the physis. Transphyseal tunnels violating 7% to 9% of the cross-sectional area of the physis in rabbits resulted in a permanent growth disturbance, whereas smaller defects of 3% to 4% did not.[24,25] Together, these animal studies suggest

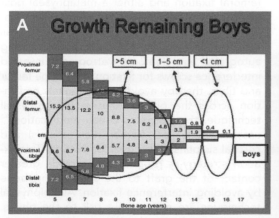
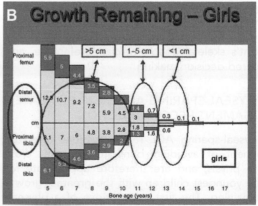

Fig. 1. Growth remaining of the distal femur and proximal tibia based on a patient's bone age: (*A*) for boys and (*B*) for girls. (*From* Perkins CA, Willimon SC, Busch MT. Transphyseal ACL Reconstruction in Skeletally Immature Patients. In: Parikh SN, editor. The Pediatric Anterior Cruciate Ligament: Evaluation and Management Strategies, 1st edition. Cham: Springer International Publishing AG; 2018; with permission.)

that soft tissue grafts placed in transphyseal tunnels across less than 5% of the cross-sectional area of the physis prevent formation of physeal bars; however, tethering may explain occasional angular deformities about the knee.[26]

Radiograph-based computer models have tried to evaluate tunnel characteristics across open physes. Kercher and colleagues[27] obtained 3-dimensional models of the physes from patients with an ACL tear on MRI. By mapping 8-mm tunnels, these investigators calculated a violation of 2.4% of the distal femoral and 2.5% of the proximal tibial physes.[27] Using a similar 3-dimensional modeling technique, Shea and associates[28] found that increasing the tibial tunnel drill angle from 45° to 70° from the horizontal decreases volume removed from 4.1% to 3.1%. However, the benefits of damaging less physis by using vertical tunnels have to be weighed against the detrimental biomechanical effects of these less anatomic and physiologic reconstructions.

OPERATIVE TREATMENT

There have been numerous studies that compare outcomes of operative and nonoperative treatment of ACL injuries in skeletally immature patients.[6,29–35] A systematic review and meta-analysis published in 2013 showed dramatic benefit to early operative management.[36] Symptoms of instability were reduced from 75% to 14%, the incidence of medial meniscal tears was reduced from 35% to 4%, and the ability to return to sports increased from 0% to 86% with timely reconstruction. As a result, operative treatment, rather than nonoperative treatment, is considered the standard of care in even the youngest athletes with an ACL injury. Physeal-sparing (extraphyseal and all-epiphyseal), partial transphyseal, and transphyseal reconstructions are all acceptable techniques based on the patient's skeletal age, physician preference, and shared decision making.

PHYSEAL-SPARING ANTERIOR CRUCIATE LIGAMENT RECONSTRUCTION

Physeal-sparing ACL reconstructions offer the benefit of avoiding bone tunnels that cross the physis, and are therefore appropriate for the youngest children with the greatest growth remaining. The first descriptions of a physeal-sparing technique were by David MacIntosh and associates[37] in 1976, who developed an extra-articular reconstruction using an iliotibial band autograft for chronic ACL deficiency in adults. The graft was harvested proximally, left intact at Gerdy's tubercle, passed deep to the fibular collateral ligament, and sutured back to itself. Micheli and colleagues[38] later described a modification of this technique to include a combined extra-articular and intra-articular reconstruction as a physeal-sparing reconstruction in skeletally immature children and adolescents. The iliotibial band is passed superficial to the fibular collateral ligament to an over-the-top position on the femur, through the intercondylar notch, beneath the intermeniscal ligament, and then sutured to the periosteum of the proximal tibia and lateral femur.[38] Although cited by some as a nonanatomic reconstruction, biomechanical testing has shown restoration of native constraint[39] and clinical outcomes cite low revision rates with this technique.[40–42]

ALL-EPIPHYSEAL ANTERIOR CRUCIATE LIGAMENT RECONSTRUCTION

All-epiphyseal ACL reconstructions offer similar benefits to the physeal-sparing iliotibial band reconstruction, but with the advantage of restoring the anatomic footprint of the ACL. Biomechanical testing of this technique demonstrates restoration of normal knee kinematics, while also decreasing the posterior joint contact stress as compared with the ACL-deficient knee.[39,43] Several all-epiphyseal ACL reconstruction techniques have been described, including the Anderson,[44] Ganley-Lawrence,[45] and Cordasco-Green,[46] each with unique tunnel drilling and fixation techniques. The Anderson technique[44] was described in 2004 and features outside-in epiphyseal bone tunnels, a quadrupled hamstring autograft, and suspensory femoral fixation and either a metaphyseal post or epiphyseal suspensory device for tibial fixation. The Ganley-Lawrence technique[45] was described in 2010, uses a quadrupled hamstring autograft, and features retrograde inserted interference screws for fixation in both the femur and tibia, thereby avoiding any tunnels or fixation across the physis. Another all-epiphyseal technique, the Cordasco-Green modification,[46] uses bone sockets (rather than tunnels) and cortical suspensory buttons for fixation. This fixation strategy is proposed to provide greater contact of the graft to the surrounding bone by avoiding interference fixation. All-epiphyseal techniques are not without risk to the physis. Lawrence and coworkers[47] reported a premature lateral distal femoral physeal closure associated with an all-epiphyseal femoral tunnel, potentially secondary to thermal injury from tunnel drilling. In contrast, other authors have described overgrowth resulting in leg-length discrepancy requiring subsequent guided growth following an all-epiphyseal tunnel, hypothesizing that the increased vascularity after periosteal disruption stimulated the increased growth of the surgical limb.[48,49] Cruz and colleagues[50] reviewed a single-center series of 103 patients treated with all-epiphyseal ACL reconstructions and identified an overall complication rate of 16.5%, including 11 graft ruptures, 1 leg-length discrepancy of greater than 1 cm, 2 cases of arthrofibrosis requiring manipulation under anesthesia, and 3 patients with subsequent ipsilateral meniscus tears. These complications raise concerns that all-epiphyseal ACL reconstructions are not without risk in patients with growth remaining.

All-epiphyseal reconstructions are growing in popularity for very young patients, but require long-term outcome studies with close follow-up for this relatively rare group of very young patients with ACL tears.

PARTIAL TRANSPHYSEAL ANTERIOR CRUCIATE LIGAMENT RECONSTRUCTION

Partial transphyseal ACL reconstructions were described as early as 1986 with over-the-top physeal-sparing femoral graft fixation and a transphyseal tibial tunnel.[51] Several other authors have described a similar over-the-top femoral graft position and a transphyseal tibial tunnel.[52,53] More recently, Milewski and Nissen[54] have described an all-epiphyseal femoral tunnel and a transphyseal tibial tunnel to allow for a more anatomic femoral tunnel position. For patients with 3 or more years of growth remaining, a partial transphyseal reconstruction offers the ability to avoid injury of the femoral physis while drilling a tibial tunnel, which is vertical and small with limited impact on the tibial physis. There are very limited outcome data for partial transphyseal ACL reconstructions. Chambers and colleagues[55] recently reported on 24 patients with a mean age of 12.3 years who underwent partial transphyseal ACL reconstruction with a hamstring autograft. The majority of patients had 2 to 5 years of growth remaining, which they defined as females with a chronologic age of 9 to 12 years and males with a chronologic age of 11 to 14 years. Mean graft size was 7.8 mm (range, 7–9 mm). Five patients (21%) experienced a growth disturbance, with 3 patients having a greater than 1 cm limb length discrepancy and 3 patients developing genu valgum. Most notable, was that of the 3

patients in the cohort with more than 5 years of growth remaining, 2 (67%) had a growth disturbance. There were 2 graft failures (8%) at a mean of 31 months of follow-up. Clearly, the youngest children with ACL tears may not be appropriate for this partial transphyseal technique. Future studies using bone age to predict growth remaining with functional outcomes will be necessary to determine the particular age group that is best treated with a partial transphyseal technique.

TRANSPHYSEAL ANTERIOR CRUCIATE LIGAMENT RECONSTRUCTION

The vast majority of ACL tears in skeletally immature athletes occur in adolescents with limited growth remaining (<1 year). This allows for traditional transphyseal reconstructions with little risk for growth disturbance. With careful patient selection and attention to technical details, a transphyseal ACL reconstruction is a sound and viable treatment for most skeletally immature children.

A survey of the Herodicus Society and ACL study group was published by Kocher and colleagues[56] in 2002 and aimed to describe cases of growth disturbances resulting from ACL reconstruction in skeletally immature children. Among 140 surgeons, there were 15 growth disturbances reported, with 12 of these occurring after transphyseal reconstructions. Of these, 3 had hardware crossing the distal femoral physes and 4 had patellar tendon bone plugs crossing a physis, resulting in premature physeal closure and angular deformity. Two patients developed limb length inequalities, one associated with a 12-mm femoral tunnel and the other with a patellar tendon bone plug crossing the physis. The final 3 patients developed recurvatum associated with staples across the tibial tubercle and multiple sutures into the periosteum of the tibia. These technical flaws highlight the importance of a physeal respecting transphyseal reconstruction.

Shiflett and coworkers[26] published a report on 4 skeletally immature patients (ages at surgery 13.5–14.8 years) with growth arrest after transphyseal ACL reconstruction with a hamstring autograft. Two patients developed tibial recurvatum with closure of the tibial apophysis and 2 patients developed genu valgum. The authors postulated that the recurvatum occurred as a result of tenoepiphysiodesis, whereby excessive tensioning of the graft across the physis at the time of a rapid growth spurt led to tibial apophysis arrest. The etiology of the distal femoral arrests resulting in genu valgum was postulated to be the oblique trajectory of the femoral tunnel created through an antero-medial portal. Despite the use of soft tissue grafts with theoretically limited injury to the physes, this report reinforces that problems can occur, transphyseal ACL reconstruction in immature youths is not yet risk free, and these patients must be followed closely to skeletal maturity. However, the vast majority of studies of transphyseal reconstruction describe favorable outcomes with no significant length or angular deformities.[33,57–64]

AUTHORS' PREFERRED APPROACH

By using Dimeglio's growth remaining data[22] (see Fig. 1), the authors have divided children undergoing ACL reconstruction into 3 treatment groups that arguably have clinical implications (Table 1). Patients with less than 1 cm of growth remaining at the knee have virtually no risk of developing a meaningful growth disturbance. These are typically males with a bone age of 15 or 16 years and females with a bone age of 13 or 14 years. In this group of patients, we feel a transphyseal reconstruction is safe. Families can be counseled that complete or partial growth arrests with minimal growth remaining have not been demonstrated to cause significant deformity. As a result, conventional ACL reconstruction techniques and graft options can be considered with minimal to no modifications. Specifically, grafts that include bone blocks, such as patellar tendon or quadriceps grafts, can be used. These patients are followed clinically for at least 12 months and discharged once radiographs show that their physes surrounding the knee have closed. Alignment is followed clinically and long leg radiographs for limb alignment are not routinely obtained.

For those patients with 1 to 5 cm of growth remaining, who have a risk of developing an

Table 1
Growth-based surgical strategy

Growth (cm)	Girls	Boys	Prescription
<1	≥13	≥15	Standard procedure
1–5	11–12	13–14	Transphyseal
>5	≤10	≤12	Physeal sparing

From Perkins CA, Willimon SC, Busch MT. Transphyseal ACL Reconstruction in Skeletally Immature Patients. In: Parikh SN, editor. The Pediatric Anterior Cruciate Ligament: Evaluation and Management Strategies, 1st edition. Cham: Springer International Publishing AG; 2018; with permission.

appreciable growth disturbance, there are several considerations that guide treatment. These are typically males with a bone age of 13 or 14 years and females with a bone age of 11 or 12 years. For them, a thoughtfully performed physeal-respecting transphyseal reconstruction is a viable option, and is our usual recommendation. Preoperatively, a left hand bone age and long leg alignment radiographs are obtained. Occasionally, we identify an existing coronal plane deformity, typically genu valgum, which may have contributed to the original ACL injury and be a risk factor for subsequent graft injury. Correction with hemi-epiphyseal tethering and guided growth can be considered.

A soft tissue autograft is selected for this age group, with the most common graft being a quadriceps tendon in our practice. Tunnels are sized according to the diameter of the graft and positioned centrally in the physis. There is mixed literature regarding optimal graft size in adolescents, but if patients are approaching adult body habitus, we strive for a graft size of 8 to 9 mm. Graft fixation is performed on the femur using cortical suspensory fixation (through a femoral tunnel drilled using a tibial independent drilling technique) and a biocomposite interference screw or post placed distal to the physis on the tibia. Fixation placement is verified with fluoroscopy. Distal fixation can be supplemented with a staple, post and washer, or anchor as deemed necessary. Careful placement of the tibial tunnel and fixation is needed to avoid additional risk of damage to the tibial tubercle and perichondral tissue.

Patients and families are advised of the risks of growth disturbance associated with this technique, but are reassured that reasonable precautions will be taken to minimize these risks and the patients will be monitored afterward to identify any growth-related abnormality. If necessary, treatment can be undertaken in a timely manner to diminish the effect of the growth disturbance and minimize the need for future interventions. Postoperatively, the examination of limb lengths and alignments is documented at each visit. If we have a clinical concern for length or angular deformities, then lower extremity alignment radiographs are obtained and may be compared with preoperative limb alignment radiographs.

For patients with more than 5 cm of growth remaining, the consequences of a growth disturbance are more significant given the amount of growth remaining. Therefore, we recommend a physeal-sparing reconstruction. This patient group typically includes males with a bone age of 12 years or less and females with a bone age of 10 years or less. In our hands, this is most commonly the iliotibial band reconstruction modified by Micheli[40] and published by Micheli, Kocher, and others.[40–42] This technique has produced good results in our practice with low failure rates and no apparent growth disturbances in our youngest patients.

REHABILITATION

In addition to careful surgical technique, a structured rehabilitation program with experienced physical therapists is important to ensure optimal outcomes after ACL reconstruction. Standard rehabilitation protocols include progressive strengthening, proprioception, and endurance. A functional testing regimen is completed at 6 months postsurgery to guide us in advancing patients to the last 3 months of a return to sport progression. Return to unrestricted cutting and pivoting sports is routinely no sooner than 9 months. This schedule is supported by reduced reinjury rates for each month that return to sports is delayed until 9 months after surgery.[65] Ultimately, a return to sport progression is guided by a combination of surgeon discretion and functional testing results. Full clearance is not provided until functional testing demonstrates safe landing mechanics and appropriate neuromuscular control, and may require 12 months or longer to achieve. Establishing clear patient and family expectations regarding restrictions and estimated return to play is critical to successful outcomes and maximizing compliance and should be a routine part of the preoperative discussion.

SUMMARY

The increasing incidence of ACL injuries in skeletally immature children demands careful attention by orthopaedic surgeons. In addition to chronologic age, assessment of skeletal age is essential to select the appropriate ACL reconstruction technique. Males with a bone age of 15 years or older and females of 13 years and older are ideal candidates for a transphyseal ACL reconstruction. Families can be reassured that there is minimal risk of growth disturbance in this age group, and few additional considerations are required for an optimal outcome.

Based on the current evidence, transphyseal ACL reconstructions with soft tissue grafts are relatively safe and effective for skeletally immature adolescents whose skeletal age is 13 or 14 years in males and 11 or 12 years in females. In this population, the risk for limb length discrepancy and angular deformity is low, but requires assessment, planning, informed consent, documentation, a physeal-respecting surgical technique, and appropriate follow-up. Children with substantial growth remaining (skeletal age boys 12 years or less and girls 10 years or less) seem to be at risk for greater significant growth disturbance, so we generally recommend physeal-sparing techniques for these younger patients.

REFERENCES

1. Comstock RD, Collins CL, McIlvain NM. Summary report: national high school sports -related injury surveillance study. 2009-2010 school year. Available at: http://www.nationwidechildrens.org/Document/Get/103353 Accessed February 1, 2019.
2. Buller LT, Best MJ, Baraga MG. Trends in anterior cruciate ligament reconstruction in the United States. Orthop J Sports Med 2015;3(1). 2325967114563664.
3. Gornitzky AL, Lott A, Yellin JL, et al. Sport-specific yearly risk and incidence of anterior cruciate ligament tears in high school athletes: a systematic review and meta-analysis. Am J Sports Med 2015;44(10):2716–23.
4. Mall NA, Paletta GA. Pediatric ACL injuries: evaluation and management. Curr Rev Musculoskelet Med 2013;6(2):132–40.
5. Lawrence JT, Argawal N, Ganley TJ. Degeneration of the knee joint in skeletally immature patients with a diagnosis of an anterior cruciate ligament tear: is there harm in delay of treatment? Am J Sports Med 2011;39(12):2582–7.
6. Millett PJ, Willis AA, Warren RF. Associated injuries in pediatric and adolescent anterior cruciate ligament tears: does a delay in treatment increase the risk of meniscal tear? Arthroscopy 2002;18(9):955–9.
7. Li G, DeFrate LE, Sun H, et al. In vivo elongation of the anterior cruciate ligament and posterior cruciate ligament during knee flexion. Am J Sports Med 2004;32(6):1415–20.
8. Ferretti M, Levicoff EA, Macpherson TA, et al. The fetal anterior cruciate ligament: an anatomic and histologic study. Arthroscopy 2007;23(3):278–83.
9. Ferretti M, Ekdahl M, Shen W, et al. Osseous landmarks of the femoral attachment of the anterior cruciate ligament: an anatomic study. Arthroscopy 2007;23(11):1218–25.
10. Girgis FG, Marshall JL, Monajem A. The cruciate ligaments of the knee joint. Anatomical, functional, and experimental analysis. Clin Orthop Relat Res 1975;106:216–31.

11. Behr CT, Potter HG, Paletta GA. The relationship of the femoral origin of the anterior cruciate ligament and the distal femoral physeal plate in the skeletally immature knee. An anatomic study. Am J Sports Med 2001;29(6):781–7.

12. Shea KG, Apel PJ, Pfeiffer RP, et al. The tibial attachment of the anterior cruciate ligament in children and adolescents: analysis of magnetic resonance imaging. Knee Surg Sports Traumatol Arthrosc 2002;10(2):102–8.

13. Shea KG, Cannamela PC, Fabricant PD, et al. Lateral radiographic landmarks for ACL and LCL footprint origins during all-epiphyseal femoral drilling in skeletally immature knees. J Bone Joint Surg Am 2017;99(6):506–11.

14. Noyes FR, Bassett RW, Grood ES, et al. Arthroscopy in acute traumatic hemarthrosis of the knee. Incidence of anterior cruciate tears and other injuries. J Bone Joint Surg Am 1980;62(5):687–95.

15. Marshall WA, Tanner JM. Variations in the pattern of pubertal changes in girls. Arch Dis Child 1969;44:291–303.

16. Slough JM, Hennrikus W, Chang Y. Reliability of Tanner staging performed by orthopedic sports medicine surgeons. Med Sci Sports Exerc 2013;45(7):1229–34.

17. Stanitski CL, Harvell JC, Fu F. Observations on acute knee hemarthrosis in children and adolescents. J Pediatr Orthop 1993;13(4):506–10.

18. Gruelich WW, Pyle SI. Radiographic atlas of skeletal development of the hand and wrist. 2nd edition. Stanford (CA): Stanford University Press; 1959.

19. Heyworth BE, Osei DA, Fabricant PD, et al. The shorthand bone age assessment: a simpler alternative to current methods. J Pediatr Orthop 2013;33(5):569–74.

20. Frank JS, Gambacorta PL. Anterior cruciate ligament injuries in the skeletally immature athlete: diagnosis and management. J Am Acad Orthop Surg 2013;21:78–87.

21. Guzzanti V, Falciglia F, Stanitski CL. Preoperative evaluation and anterior cruciate ligament reconstruction technique for skeletally immature patients in tanner stages 2 and 3. Am J Sports Med 2003;31(6):941–8.

22. Kelly PM, Dimeglio A. Lower-limb growth: how predictable are predictions? J Child Orthop 2008;2:407–15.

23. Campbell CJ, Grisolia A, Zanconato G. The effects produced in the cartilaginous epiphyseal plate of immature dogs by experimental surgical trauma. J Bone Joint Surg Am 1959;41(7):1221–42.

24. Janarv PM, Wikstrom B, Hirsch G. The influence of transphyseal drilling and tendon grafting on bone growth: an experimental study in the rabbit. J Pediatr Orthop 1998;18(2):149–54.

25. Makela EA, Vainionpaa S, Vihtonen K, et al. The effect of trauma to the lower femoral epiphyseal plate: an experimental study in rabbits. J Bone Joint Surg Br 1988;70:187–91.

26. Shiflett GD, Green DW, Widmann RF, et al. Growth arrest following ACL reconstruction with hamstring autograft in skeletally immature patients. A review of 4 cases. J Pediatr Orthop 2016;36(4):355–61.

27. Kercher J, Xerogeanes J, Tannenbaum A, et al. Anterior cruciate ligament reconstruction in the skeletally immature: an anatomical study utilizing 3-dimensional magnetic resonance imaging reconstructions. J Pediatr Orthop 2009;29(2):124–9.

28. Shea KG, Apel PJ, Pfeiffer RP. Anterior cruciate ligament injury in paediatric and adolescent patients: a review of basic science and clinical research. Sports Med 2003;33:455–71.

29. Graf BK, Lange RH, Fujisaki CK, et al. Anterior cruciate ligament tears in skeletally immature patients: meniscal pathology at presentation and after attempted conservative treatment. Arthroscopy 1992;8(2):229–33.

30. Henry J, Chotel F, Chouteau J, et al. Rupture of the anterior cruciate ligament in children: early reconstruction with open physes or delayed reconstruction to skeletal maturity? Knee Surg Sports Traumatol Arthrosc 2009;17(7):748–55.

31. Janarv PM, Nystrom A, Werner S, et al. Anterior cruciate ligament injuries in skeletally immature patients. J Pediatr Orthop 1996;16(5):673–7.

32. McCarroll JR, Rettig AC, Shelbourne KD. Anterior cruciate ligament injuries in the young athlete with open physes. Am J Sports Med 1988;16(1):44–7.

33. Pressman AE, Letts RM, Jarvis JG. Anterior cruciate ligament tears in children: an analysis of operative versus nonoperative treatment. J Pediatr Orthop 1997;17(4):505–11.

34. Streich NA, Barie A, Gotterbarm T, et al. Transphyseal reconstruction of the anterior cruciate ligament in prepubescent athletes. Knee Surg Sports Traumatol Arthrosc 2010;18(11):1481–6.

35. Woods GW, O'Connor DP. Delayed anterior cruciate ligament reconstruction in adolescents with open physes. Am J Sports Med 2004;32(1):201–10.

36. Ramski DE, Kanj WW, Franklin CC, et al. Anterior cruciate ligament tears in children and adolescents: a meta-analysis of nonoperative versus operative treatment. Am J Sports Med 2014;42(11):2769–76.

37. MacIntosh DL, Darby TA. Lateral substitution reconstruction. In: Proceedings of the Canadian orthopaedic association. J Bone Joint Surg 1976;1:142.

38. Micheli LJ, Rask B, Gerberg L. Anterior cruciate ligament reconstruction in patients who are prepubescent. Clin Orthop Relat Res 1999;364:40–7.

39. Kennedy A, Coughlin DG, Metzger MF, et al. Biomechanical evaluation of pediatric anterior

cruciate ligament reconstruction techniques. Am J Sports Med 2011;39(5):964–71.

40. Kocher MS, Garg S, Micheli LJ. Physeal sparing reconstruction of the anterior cruciate ligament in skeletally immature prepubescent children and adolescents. J Bone Joint Surg Am 2005;11:2371–9.

41. Kocher MS, Heyworth BE, Fabricant PD, et al. Outcomes of physeal-sparing ACL reconstruction with iliotibial band autograft in skeletally immature prepubescent children. J Bone Joint Surg Am 2018; 100(13):1087–894.

42. Willimon SC, Jones CR, Herzog MM, et al. Micheli anterior cruciate ligament reconstruction in skeletally immature youths: a retrospective case series with a mean 3-year follow-up. Am J Sports Med 2015;43(12):2974–81.

43. McCarthy MM, Tucker S, Nguyen JT, et al. Contact stress and kinematic analysis of all-epiphyseal and over-the-top pediatric reconstruction techniques for the anterior cruciate ligament. Am J Sports Med 2013;41(6):1330–9.

44. Anderson AF. Transepiphyseal replacement of the anterior cruciate ligament using quadruple hamstring grafts in skeletally immature patients. J Bone Joint Surg Am 2004;86:201–9.

45. Lawrence JT, Bowers AL, Belding J, et al. All-epiphyseal anterior cruciate ligament reconstruction in skeletally immature patients. Clin Orthop Relat Res 2010;468(7):1971–7.

46. McCarthy MM, Graziano J, Green DW, et al. All-epiphyseal, all-inside anterior cruciate ligament reconstruction technique for skeletally immature patients. Arthrosc Tech 2012;1(2):231–9.

47. Lawrence JT, West RL, Garrett WE. Growth disturbance following ACL reconstruction with use of an epiphyseal femoral tunnel: a case report. J Bone Joint Surg Am 2011;93(8):39.

48. Koch PP, Fucentese SF, Blatter SC. Complications after epiphyseal reconstruction of the anterior cruciate ligament in prepubescent children. Knee Surg Sports Traumatol Arthrosc 2016;24(9):2736–40.

49. Wall EJ, Ghattas PJ, Eismann EA, et al. Outcomes and complications after all-epiphyseal anterior cruciate ligament reconstruction in skeletally immature patients. Orthop J Sports Med 2017; 5(3). 2325967117693604.

50. Cruz AI, Fabricant PD, McGraw M, et al. All-epiphyseal ACL reconstruction in children: review of safety and early complications. J Pediatr Orthop 2017;37(3):204–9.

51. Lipscomb AB, Anderson AF. Tears of the anterior cruciate ligament in adolescents. J Bone Joint Surg Am 1986;68:19–28.

52. Andrews M, Noyes F, Barber-Westin SD. Anterior cruciate ligament allograft reconstruction in the skeletally immature athlete. Am J Sports Med 1994;22:48–54.

53. Lo IK, Kirkley A, Fowler PJ, et al. The outcome of operatively treated anterior cruciate ligament disruptions in the skeletally immature child. Arthroscopy 1997;13:627–34.

54. Milewski MD, Nissen CW. Femoral physeal sparing/transphyseal tibia (hybrid) technique for ACL reconstruction in skeletally immature athletes. In: Parikh SN, editor. The pediatric anterior cruciate ligament. Switzerland: Springer Cham; 2018. p. 147–55.

55. Chambers CC, Monroe EJ, Allen CR, et al. Partial transphyseal anterior cruciate ligament reconstruction: clinical, functional, and radiographic outcomes. Am J Sports Med 2019;47(6).

56. Kocher MS, Saxon HS, Hovis WD, et al. Management and complications of anterior cruciate ligament injuries in skeletally immature patients: survey of The Herodicus Society and the ACL Study Group. J Pediatr Orthop 2002;22:452–7.

57. Aichroth PM, Patel DV, Zorrilla P. The natural history and treatment of rupture of the anterior cruciate ligament in children and adolescents: a prospective review. J Bone Joint Surg Br 2002;84:38–41.

58. Calvo R, Figueroa D, Gili F, et al. Transphyseal anterior cruciate ligament reconstruction in patients with open physes: 10-year follow-up study. Am J Sports Med 2015;43(2):289–94.

59. Kim SJ, Shim DW, Park KW. Functional outcome of transphyseal reconstruction of the anterior cruciate ligament in skeletally immature patients. Knee Surg Relat Res 2012;24(3):173–9.

60. Kocher MS, Smith JT, Zoric JB, et al. Transphyseal anterior cruciate ligament reconstruction in skeletally immature pubescent adolescents. J Bone Joint Surg Am 2007;89(12):2632–9.

61. Kohl S, Stutz C, Decker S, et al. Mid-term results of transphyseal anterior cruciate ligament reconstruction in children and adolescents. Knee 2014;21(1): 80–5.

62. Liddle AD, Imbuldeniya AM, Hunt DM. Transphyseal reconstruction of the anterior cruciate ligament in prepubescent children. J Bone Joint Surg Br 2008;90(10):1317–22.

63. Redler LH, Brafman RT, Trentacosta N, et al. Anterior cruciate ligament reconstruction in skeletally immature patients with transphyseal tunnels. Arthroscopy 2012;28(11):1710–7.

64. Shelbourne KD, Gray T, Wiley BV. Results of transphyseal anterior cruciate ligament reconstruction using patellar tendon autograft in tanner stage 3 or 4 adolescents with clearly open growth plates. Am J Sports Med 2004;32(5):1218–22.

65. Grindem H, Snyder-Mackler L, Moksnes H, et al. Simple decision rules reduce reinjury risk after anterior cruciate ligament reconstruction. The Delaware-Oslo ACL cohort study. Br J Sports Med 2016;50(13):804–8.

Hand and Wrist

Scaphoid Reconstruction

Cristian S. Borges, MD[a,b,*], Paulo H. Ruschel, MD[a,b],
Milton B. Pignataro, MD[a,b]

KEYWORDS

• Scaphoid • Nonunion • Bone graft • SNAC wrist • Bone reconstruction

KEY POINTS

- Surgical strategies for scaphoid nonunions often become more complex based on the time from injury to treatment; the decision-making process, however, can follow a logical sequence.
- Scaphoid nonunions with less than 1 year after trauma and no carpal malalignment can be treated with percutaneous screw fixation under fluoroscopic and/or arthroscopic guidance.
- Resection of the distal pole of the scaphoid is a good option in old (>5 year old) or after failed scaphoid procedure in selected patients.
- When there is radioscaphoid degenerative changes, salvage procedures like proximal row carpectomy or partial wrist fusions should be considered.
- The authors' preference is for proximal row carpectomy because the technique is simpler, immobilization periods shorter, complications fewer, and outcomes similar or superior to more complex interventions.

INTRODUCTION

The scaphoid is the most commonly fractured carpal bone, accounting for 60% of the fractures in the carpus. Up to 33% of those fractures are not seen on plain radiographs in the emergency department.[1] Approximately 10% of fractures in scaphoid fail to consolidate despite adequate immobilization.[2–4] The scaphoid has many particular characteristics that make it prone to nonunion and an unsuccessful outcome. Eighty percent of the scaphoid surface is covered by cartilage, and 70% to 80% of the blood supply to the scaphoid is provided by branches of the radial artery entering at the dorsal ridge in a predominantly retrograde manner.[5] The scaphoid is a link between the proximal and distal carpal rows and is subject to significant forces that lead to a tendency for flexion and shortening of the bone fragments.[6]

Besides the intrinsic characteristics that make scaphoid fractures prone to nonunion, risk factors for scaphoid nonunion are well-known: location of scaphoid fracture (proximal third),

fracture displacement, carpal instability, time to treatment, heavy labor, and smoking.[4]

Scaphoid fractures that do not show signs of healing 6 months after the traumatic event are considered as nonunions.[4,7] Some authors even consider 3 to 4 months of lack of progression toward healing as delayed union or nonunion.[4,8]

Scaphoid nonunion has a predictable outcome. Bone resorption and fragment displacement lead to flexion and shortening of the scaphoid. Dorsal prominence at the nonunion site can cause a humpback deformity that has a tendency to impinge on the dorsal rim of the distal radius scaphoid fossa. Displaced scaphoid fragments lead to a nondissociative instability pattern and radioscaphoid incongruence leading to radiocarpal joint osteoarthritic changes that progresses from the radial styloid process to scaphoid fossa and then to midcarpal joint and lunate fossa. All these changes lead to pain and restrictions in the range of motion. The purpose of scaphoid reconstruction is to restore length, carpal alignment, and kinematics and to prevent further progression of cartilage

[a] Division of the Orthopedics and Traumatology Department, Santa Casa Hospital Complex, Porto Alegre, Brazil;
[b] Clinica da Mao ao Cotovelo, 569/601 Soledade Street, Porto Alegre, Rio Grande do Sul 90470-340, Brazil
* Corresponding author. Clinica da Mao ao Cotovelo. 569/601 Soledade Street. Porto Alegre, Rio Grande do Sul 90470-340, Brazil.
E-mail address: steinborges5@gmail.com

Orthop Clin N Am 51 (2020) 65–76
https://doi.org/10.1016/j.ocl.2019.08.010
0030-5898/20/© 2019 Elsevier Inc. All rights reserved.

degeneration.[4] This article addresses the management of scaphoid fractures in skeletally mature patients.

SCAPHOID NONUNION WITH NO CARPAL MALALIGNMENT

Slade and Dodds[9] proposed a 6-grade system that uses anatomic and physiologic features. Several authors have based their treatment algorithms on this system. Scaphoid nonunions that have no bone loss, have viable bone fragments, and have no carpal malalignment can be reliably treated with a minimally invasive approach with percutaneous fixation with or without arthroscopic assistance. There are many advantages to this approach: no donor site morbidity, less time consuming, technically less demanding, less disturbance of scaphoid vascularity, and less surgically invasive (Table 1).

Slade and colleagues[10] popularized the concept of treating selected cases of scaphoid nonunion with percutaneous fixation and no grafting after a publication of a series of 15 patients. The author achieved union in all patients as seen on computed tomography (CT) scans and achieved 12 excellent and 3 good results based on the Mayo modified wrist score.

Slade and Gillon[11] published a consecutive series of 234 scaphoid fracture nonunions treated with arthroscopically assisted percutaneous fixation. One hundred eight cases were in the nonunion group (10 cases failed to heal and had to be reoperated). The authors concluded that this method was effective and safe for scaphoid nonunions.

Arthroscopic assistance for percutaneous fixation demands significant experience with arthroscopic procedures, but allows the surgeon to have a better assessment of the concomitant lesions that might be present at the wrist joint. Many authors have presented case series with successful outcomes with percutaneous fixation under fluoroscopic guidance only.

Capo and colleagues[12] published a series of 12 cases of scaphoid nonunions. A volar percutaneous approach was used in 8 patients and a dorsal percutaneous approach in 4 patients.

Table 1
Treatment classification system for Scaphoid nonunions

Grade	Category	Characteristics of Scaphoid Nonunions
I	Delayed presentation	Scaphoid fractures with delayed presentation (4–8 wk)
II	Fibrous nonunion	Intact cartilaginous envelope, minimal fracture line at nonunion interface, no cyst or sclerosis
III	Minimal sclerosis	Bone resorption at nonunion interface <1 mm with minimal sclerosis
IV	Cyst formation and sclerosis	Bone resorption at nonunion interface <5 mm, cyst formation, and maintained scaphoid alignment
V	Cyst formation and sclerosis	Bone resorption at nonunion interface >5 mm and <10 mm, cyst formation, and maintained scaphoid alignment
VI	Pseudoarthrosis	Separate bone fracture fragments with profound bone resorption at nonunion interface. Gross fragment motion and deformity is often present.
Subtypes	**Category**	**Associated Characteristics**
a	Proximal pole nonunion	The proximal pole has a tenuous blood supply and a mechanical disadvantage that places it at greater risk of delayed or failed union.
b	Avascular necrosis	Scaphoid nonunion with avascular necrosis confirmed by MRI or intraoperative lack of punctate bleeding. The fracture must heal and revitalize.
c	Ligamentous injury	Injury suggested by static and dynamic imaging of the carpal bones or arthroscopic, direct observation.
d	Deformity	Scaphoid deformity must be corrected. This requires a bicortical structural bone graft and rigid fixation.

From Slade JF, Dodds SD. Minimally invasive management of scaphoid nonunions. Clin Orthop Relat Res 2006;445:112; with permission.

The authors achieved a 92% union rate and good functional scores (Disabilities of the Arm, Shoulder and Hand and range of motion). One patient had revision surgery and achieved healing after percutaneous bone grafting and fixation.

Kim and colleagues[13] published their results of 12 scaphoid fractures with delayed union and nonunion. Scaphoid waist fractures with delayed union included fractures with no signs of healing after 8 weeks of cast immobilization and late fractures presenting between 4 weeks and 6 months after injury. No patient in the series had carpal instability, scaphoid deformity, or avascular necrosis of the proximal fracture fragment. All patients achieved healing, good functional outcomes, and satisfying patient-related scores.

Somerson and colleagues[14] published a series of 14 cases of scaphoid nonunions treated with percutaneous fixation and no bone grafting. Twelve of the 14 patients healed successfully, whereas 2 patients required secondary vascularized bone grafting. Both nonunion patients sustained proximal pole fractures and had a duration of 1 year or more from injury to surgery. These authors concluded that percutaneous fixation alone is a reliable method, but age and delay from injury to surgery of 1 year or more lead to poorer outcomes.

Vanhees and colleagues[15] published a retrospective study of 16 patients with delayed unions and nonunions without any previous treatment. All patients were treated with percutaneous screw fixation. At a mean of 4 months, a 94% union rate was obtained based on CT scans with good functional results on the Disabilities of the Arm, Shoulder and Hand and Patient-Rated Wrist and Hand Evaluation when there was no sclerosis, minimal osteolysis, and no displacement at the scaphoid nonunion site.

Hegazy[16] published a series of 21 cases of scaphoid nonunions treated with percutaneous screw fixation. The inclusion criteria in this series were scaphoid waist fracture nonunions with intact cartilaginous envelope, minimal fracture line at nonunion interface, no cyst or sclerosis, no avascular necrosis, and a normal scapholunate angle without humpback deformity. All fractures united successfully with no additional procedures.

Hence, the authors of this article recommend percutaneous screw fixation without bone graft in cases of scaphoid nonunions with less than 1 year after traumatic event, minimally displaced fragments (<1 mm), minimal bone resorption (<2 mm), minimal sclerosis, absence of vascular necrosis, and no humpback deformity.

Larger bone gaps can be treated with percutaneous fixation alone in selected cases. Mahmoud and Koptan[17] published a series of 27 patients with scaphoid nonunion with substantial bone loss (Slade grades IV and V). All of them achieved bone union and good functional outcomes. No patient had avascular necrosis (as seen on plain radiographs) or had a humpback deformity as seen on CT scans. The authors recommend this method of treatment for patients who are middle-aged nonsmokers without previous wrist surgery who have a scaphoid waist nonunion with no deformity, no avascular necrosis, and adequate fragments for good purchase with a cannulated screw (Fig. 1).

SCAPHOID NONUNION WITH CARPAL COLLAPSE

Scaphoid nonunions with significant bone loss and carpal malalignment (capitulolunate angle of >15°) need correction with addition of bone graft to restore length and normal intrascaphoid angle. Besides the correction of anatomic length and intrascaphoid angle, there is a need to correct the humpback deformity to prevent further impingement in the dorsal rim of the radius.

Most of the nonunions associated with bone loss and changes in length and shape of the scaphoid are located at the middle third or waist of the scaphoid. That means that usually the proximal pole is viable and large enough for a good purchase from an implant (wire, screws or plates).

The source of bone is a subject of surgeon's own preference, but the literature can shed some light on that decision. Traditionally, bone grafts from the iliac crest became more widely used based on the reports of good results in restoration of normal scaphoid anatomy.[18,19] Grafts from the iliac crest have more mechanical resistance to compressive loads and excellent osteogenic potential. Some authors challenged this concept believing that the distal radius could be a source as reliable, because the iliac crest and had the additional benefit of being available in the same operative field.[20,21]

Tambe and colleagues[22] retrospectively studied a consecutive cohort of 68 symptomatic established scaphoid nonunions treated by bone grafting. Iliac crest graft was used in 44 cases and a distal radius graft in the other 24. The 2 treatment groups were comparable in terms of location of the fracture, nonunion duration, and implant fixation. They found a 66%

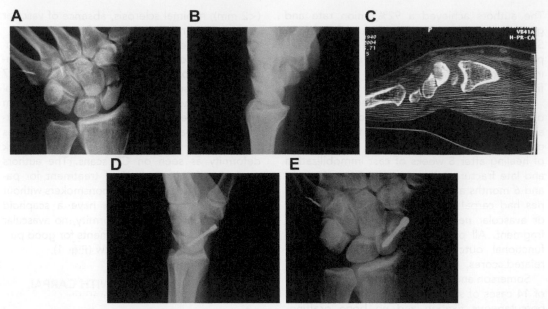

Fig. 1. (A–E) Percutaneous screw fixation with no graft. (A) Scaphoid nonunion with cyst formation but preserved length. (B) No carpal malalignment on lateral view. (C) No humpback deformity on CT scan. (D) Lateral view. (E) Posteroanterior view.

consolidation rate in the iliac graft group versus 67% in the distal radius graft group. The differences were only significant in terms of donor site persistent pain, which was much higher in the iliac crest graft group.

Garg and colleagues[23] published a prospective randomized controlled trial comparing 50 patients treated with iliac bone graft and 50 patients treated with distal radius bone graft. There was no statistically significant difference between the 2 groups in terms of range of motion, functional scores, union rate, or fracture reduction. The authors concluded that there is no advantage of the iliac crest over the distal radius graft to justify its greater morbidity.

Cancellous bone graft has the advantage over structural corticocancellous graft when osteogenic capacity is considered, but is widely regarded as structurally insufficient to provide mechanical support and maintain the anatomy of the scaphoid. Kim and colleagues[24] in a retrospective cohort study compared 17 patients with unstable scaphoid nonunion treated with corticocancellous bone graft with 18 patients treated with cancellous bone graft only. Cancellous bone grafting was found to lead to earlier bone union than corticocancellous bone grafting and to similar restorations of scaphoid deformity and wrist function when scaphoid nonunions were treated by headless compression screw fixation and crest bone grafting.

Sayegh and Strauch[25] published in 2014 a metanalysis that compiled data from 23 studies between 1987 and 2013 containing 604 patients. They compared results between cancellous only and corticocancellous bone graft for scaphoid nonunion. Corticocancellous grafts significantly improved the scapholunate and radiolunate angles more than cancellous-only grafts. Nevertheless, cancellous-only grafts provide the shortest interval to union for unstable scaphoid nonunions and are associated with consistent deformity correction and superior Mayo wrist scores.

Nonvascularized bone grafts have the advantage of being less technically demanding and time consuming. As long as there is enough bone for implant stability and viable fragments, predictable union rates and functional outcomes are expected.

Whenever proximal pole is viable as seen on MRI we have a preference for wedge-shaped corticocancellous bone and compression screw. We believe that a precise geometry of the graft and recipient site, cut precisely with an oscillating saw instead of rongeurs and curettes, increases the contact between graft and scaphoid poles, and provides extra stability.

It is a rather infrequent for scaphoid waist nonunions, which are prone to collapse in flexion and subsequent shortening to have avascular proximal poles. However, when dysvascular proximal scaphoid fragments are identified, vascularized bone grafts should be considered. It should be noted that most vascularized bone grafts are not adequate to restore scaphoid geometry when there is significant bone loss because of the restricted maximum dimensions of the bone that can be harvested.

The first vascularized bone graft used to treat scaphoid nonunion was published by Roy-Camille in 1965.[26] The author used the scaphoid tuberosity vascularized by thenar muscle attachments. A similar concept was published in 1988 by Kawai and Yamamoto[27] when they reported their results of a vascularized bone graft based on attachments of the pronator quadratus muscle.

In 1987, Kuhlmann and coworkers[28] published the first results of a vascularized bone graft harvested on the palmar-ulnar side of the radius based on the palmar carpal artery. Mathoulin and Haerle[29] later popularized the results of this technique after a report with the use of a bone graft vascularized by the palmar carpal artery for the treatment of scaphoid nonunion in 17 patients, 10 of whom had already had unsuccessful surgery. Union was obtained in all cases at an average of 60 days (range, 45–90 days).

In 1991, Zaidemberg and associates[30] published an anatomic study of a pedicled vascularized bone graft harvested from the dorsoradial wrist and a series of 11 patients with treated with such for scaphoid nonunions. All cases exhibited radiographic union. The average length of immobilization to radiographic and clinical union was 6.2 weeks. The grafts were vascularized by what was then called the ascending irrigating branch of the radial artery In 1995, Sheetz and colleagues[31] published an extensive anatomic study of the vascular supply to the distal radius and ulna and conceived many possible bone flaps. The ascending irrigating branch was renamed as the 1,2 supraretinacular artery and is widely known by this name since then. Most pedicled bone flaps studies so far are based on the technique described by Zaidemberg.

Guimberteau and Panconi in 1990[32] published a series of 11patients treated with vascularized bone graft harvested from distal ulna. In all 8 patients, primary osseous union occurred in an average of 4.6 months. All were able to resume their previous occupational or athletic activities.

Bertelli and colleagues in 2004[33] popularized the technique of bone flap reconstruction for scaphoid nonunions based on the first dorsal metacarpal artery after publishing a series of 24 cases, 15 of them with incipient radiologic

osteoarthritis. The authors achieved a 100% union rate with this method.

Sotereanos and colleagues[34] published in 2006 a series of 13 scaphoid nonunions treated with a capsular-based vascularized bone graft. Despite raising the flap in the area supposedly supplied by the fourth extensor compartment artery, the vessel dissection was not pursued during dissection. Ten of the 13 patients obtained union and 3 had persistent nonunions. The authors support the technique because of its easy dissection and no major donor site morbidity.

It is reasonable to question whether the pedicled bone grafts remain vascularized after all the intraoperative process of harvesting, carving and fixation. An interesting study published in 2019 by Antoniou and colleagues[35] identified persistent blood flow after a procedure for scaphoid nonunion with the 1,2 supraretinacular bone flap. In 13 of 14 patients, the artery was patent as seen on contrast-enhanced MRI.

Vascularized bone flaps have been compared with nonvascularized grafts by many authors. Ribak and colleagues[36] published a randomized controlled trial with 46 scaphoid nonunions treated with vascularized bone graft (Zaidemberg technique) compared with 40 nonunions treated with bone graft from the distal radius. The authors achieved an 89.1% union rate with a mean time to union of 9.7 weeks in the vascularized bone graft group compared with 72.5% union rate with a mean time to union of 12 weeks in the nonvascularized group. The authors observed better results when vascularized bone grafts were compared with nonvascularized groups in patients with avascular proximal poles.

Caporrino and colleagues[37] published a randomized controlled trial with 75 patients in 2 separate groups. One group was treated with vascularized bone graft based on the 1,2 supraretinacular artery graft and the other treated with nonvascularized graft harvested from distal radius. The authors found similar union rates and functional scores. The only significant difference was that union was achieved 12 days earlier on average in the vascularized bone group.

Pinder and colleagues[38] in a systematic review of the literature compiled the results of 48 eligible studies with a total of 1602 patients. Vascularized and nonvascularized bone grafts had an estimated union incidence of 92% and 88%, respectively. The authors recognized that, if vascularized grafts were used more often for nonunions, were more likely to fail (proximal pole and avascular necrosis) or require new vascularity; however, these figures may be skewed in favor of nonvascularized grafts.

Alluri and colleagues[39] conducted a systematic review of the literature on the use of vascularized bone grafts for scaphoid nonunion. A total of 41 publications were included in final analysis. Vascularized bone grafts had an 84.7% union rate at 13 weeks after surgery. On an average, 89% of patients returned to preinjury activity levels by 18 weeks after surgery and 91% of patients reported satisfaction with the procedure. The authors demonstrate that vascularized bone grafting as a revision procedure has similar outcomes across all metrics when compared with vascularized bone grafting done as a primary surgical intervention.

The authors of this article recognize that vascularized bone grafts are powerful tools in the treatment of scaphoid nonunions (especially as onlay bone grafts), but reserve this concept for cases with avascular proximal poles or failed previous surgery. As an onlay graft or when no correction of scaphoid anatomy is necessary, the 1,2 intercompartmental supraretinacular bone flap (Zaidemberg technique) is our preferred technique. When an inlay vascularized graft for some length restoration is considered, a palmar pedicle graft (Mathoulin technique) seems to be a better choice. We have a

preference for fixation of the grafts with small (1.5 or 2.0 mm) screws instead of Kirschner wires (Fig. 2).

SCAPHOID NONUNION WITH AVASCULAR PROXIMAL POLES

Proximal pole vascularity can be reliably assessed through MRI,[40,41] even when not enhanced by a contrast agent.[42] Theoretically, vascularized bone grafts are preferred for nonunions with avascular proximal poles. Nevertheless, some authors have achieved good results with nonvascularized grafts, even in avascular proximal poles.

Kim and colleagues[43] presented the surgical outcomes of nonvascularized bone grafting taken from the iliac crest in 24 patients with scaphoid nonunion and avascular necrosis. The Fisk-Fernandez technique was used in 11 patients, and cancellous bone grafting was used in 13 patients. Bony union was achieved in 22 of the 24 patients based on CT scan images. These authors concluded that nonvascularized bone grafting can be used for vascular proximal poles nonunion.

Putnan and colleagues[44] published a retrospective study of 13 cases of scaphoid nonunion with avascular proximal poles identified by MRI.

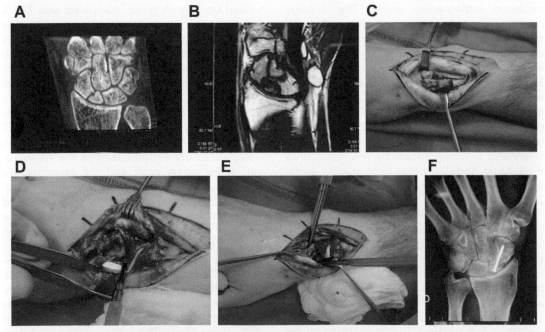

Fig. 2. (A–F) 1,2 Intercompartmental supraretinacular artery flap (1, 2 ICSRA). (A) Proximal pole as seen on CT scan. (B) MRI showing avascular proximal pole. (C) Graft being raised after 1,2 intercompartmental supraretinacular artery is dissected. (D) Recipient site prepared in the scaphoid. (E) Bone graft placed on nonunion site. (F) Postoperative radiograph showing signs of consolidation.

Patients were treated with plate fixation and pure cancellous bone grafting from the ipsilateral olecranon and/or distal radius, and application of a volar locking plate. Postoperative outcome measures included time to union based on CT scans, patient-reported pain and disability scores, grip strength, range of motion, and return to work and sports. All patients achieved bone union and good functional and patient-reported outcomes. Nevertheless, 4 patients (30%) took 24 to 30 weeks to heal.

Merrell and colleagues[4] in a meta-analysis compiled the results of the treatment of scaphoid nonunions. For avascular necrosis of the proximal fragment (seen as a lack of intraoperative punctate bleeding), union was achieved in 88% of those patients with a vascularized graft versus 47% with screw and wedge fixation.

Chang and colleagues[45] reported 50 cases of scaphoid nonunion treated with 1,2 intercompartmental supraretinacular artery bone graft. When vascularity of proximal pole was preserved, 21 of 23 cases achieved bony union. However, when proximal pole avascular necrosis was present, only 12 of 24 cases achieved bony union.

Ferguson and colleagues[46] published in 2015 a metanalysis that compiled data from 144 studies (5464 scaphoid nonunion outcomes). Mean reported union rates for vascularized and nonvascularized bone graft were 84% and 80%, respectively. The vascularized bone graft union rate was 74% compared with 62% with nonvascularized bone graft. The problem with the data from studies on patients with avascular pole necrosis in this review is that 23 of 40 reported series relied on transoperarative view or plain radiographs for the diagnosis of avascularity.

Pinder and colleagues[38] found in their meta-analysis published in 2015 union rates from 95% to 100% in the management of avascular proximal poles with vascularized bone grafts. The authors considered that improved rates when compared with the metanalysis previously (2002) published by Merrell and colleagues[4] could possibly be attributed to improvements in the management of avascular necrosis over the years.

Pedicled vascularized bone grafts are effective to improve vascularity and union rates in scaphoid nonunions with avascular proximal poles and revision surgeries. The drawback is the limited amount of bone that can be harvested in the rare circumstances when there is need to provide vascular inflow and enough bone to restore length after correction of humpback deformity and collapse of the scaphoid fragments.

There is increasing popularity of the use of free vascularized bone grafts based on medial condyle of the femur for these special cases. Doi and colleagues[47] popularized this technique after publishing a case series with 10 nonunions treated with free medial femoral condyle bone grafts based on the articular branch of the descending genicular artery. Anastomosis was performed end to side to the radial artery and end-to-end to the venae comitantes. The authors achieved a 100% union rate.

Jones and colleagues[48] published in 2010 a retrospective series of 12 patients treated with free medial femoral condyle bone grafts. The authors achieved a 100% union rate at a mean of 13 weeks. The authors found statistically significant improvement of restoration of scaphoid length and carpal alignment.

Al-Jabri and colleagues[49] published in 2014 a meta-analysis comparing 2 free vascularized bone grafts: iliac crest and medial femoral condyle. The authors compiled the results of 245 cases found in the literature. Fifty-six patients underwent free vascularized bone grafts from the medial femoral condyle with a 100% union rate and 188 patients underwent free vascularized bone grafting from the iliac crest with an 87.7% union rate. The difference between the 2 similar groups was statistically significant ($P = .006$).

Union rates of scaphoid nonunions using free medial femoral condyle grafts published so far are exceptionally optimistic. Elgammal and Lukas[50] published in 2015 a series of 30 scaphoid nonunions treated with this method and achieved 80% union rate. Still, the authors consider the union rates excellent and the capacity to restore length and vascularity provided by this technique very promising.

Some studies compared results of free medial femoral condyle with pedicle distal radius vascularized bone grafts. Jones and colleagues[51] published a retrospective series of cases of scaphoid nonunions with avascular proximal poles and carpal collapse. Ten patients were treated with 1,2 intercompartmental supraretinacular bone flaps and 12 with medial femoral condyle bone flaps. The union rate was significant higher (40% and 100%, respectively) and mean time to healing shorter (19 and 13 weeks, respectively) in the free medial condyle group.

Aibinder and colleagues[52] published a retrospective review of scaphoid nonunions treated with bone graft interposition. Thirty-one patients had corticocancellous graft from iliac crest, 33 patients had vascularized graft based on 1,2 intercompartmental supraretinacular artery and 45 patients were treated with a free medial femoral condyle flap. Union rates and mean time to union were 71% and 19 weeks for the iliac bone crest group, 79% and 26 weeks for the 1,2-intercompartmental supraretinacular artery group, and 89% and 16 weeks for the free medial femoral condyle flap group, respectively. Failure of union was associated with tobacco use but not with age, gender, time from injury to surgery, or type of fixation. There was no significant difference between the groups regarding range of motion or strength.

The free medial femoral condyle flap is a technically demanding procedure with a relatively extensive dissection and some concerns concerning morbidity may be raised. Addressing this topic, Windhofer and colleagues[53] retrospectively reviewed 45 patients and found minimal donor site morbidity. Although 21 patients could not be reached most of the patients had limited symptoms.

The free medial femoral condyle bone flap is our graft of choice in the rare circumstance of proximal pole avascular necrosis or failed prior reconstruction and carpal collapse. We

routinely look for a perforator to the skin as a monitor and as a strategy to close the skin without tension over the anastomosis (Fig. 3).

SALVAGE PROCEDURES

Scaphoid reconstruction can be considered as long there are reliable cartilage surfaces in the radiocarpal joint, the scaphoid, or both. When this essential condition is not satisfied, some other strategies should be adopted. Some old nonunions (>5 years from trauma) may be better treated not with reconstruction, but rather salvage procedures. Salvage procedures generally include radial styloidectomy, distal scaphoid resection, proximal row carpectomy (PRC), scaphoid excision and intercarpal arthrodesis, and total wrist arthrodesis.

Radial styloidectomy can be considered in early stage scaphoid nonunion advanced collapse.[54] Rarely is radial styloidectomy performed as an isolated procedure; more often, it is used as an adjunct to scaphoid reconstruction or PRC and limited intercarpal arthrodesis techniques. A radial styloidectomy can provide some relief especially in radial deviation. But

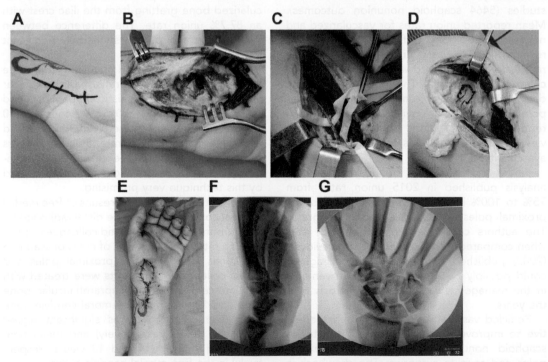

Fig. 3. (A–G) Scaphoid reconstruction with free medial femoral bone flap (MCF). (A) Skin incision. (B) Nonunion site, prepared with oscillating saw and isolation of radial artery and 2 venae comitantes. (C) Donor site dissection. Note in the upper left quadrant of the figure the design of the skin flap based on perforator probed by a portable Doppler ultrasound imaging. (D) Skin monitor and graft design. (E) Flap placed in the planned position after fixation and anastomosis. (F, G) Posteroanterior and lateral views of scaphoid reconstructed with MCF.

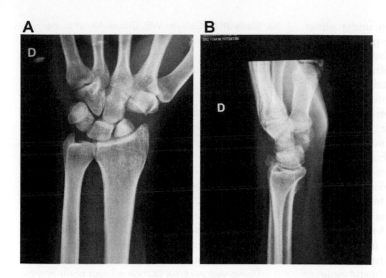

Fig. 4. (*A, B*) Resection of the distal pole of the scaphoid. A dorsal intercalated segment instability (DISI) pattern may develop, but with no major clinical implications.

only when osteoarthritis has not progressed to proximal radioscaphoid joint.

Partial wrist denervation such as distal anterior and posterior interosseous neurectomy can be considered in selected patients as an isolated limited surgical strategy or more commonly used as adjuncts to wrist salvage procedures. Despite some concerns about damage to proprioception, no clinical relevance of that impairment has been demonstrated.[55]

A simple and effective strategy for the treatment of failed or old (>5 years) scaphoid nonunions is distal scaphoid pole excision. The main indication is for patients with symptomatic wrist extension and radial deviation impingement with hypertrophic distal scaphoid poles. Malerich and colleagues[56] published in 2014 a retrospective case series (19 patients) with mean follow-up of 15 years regarding resection of the distal pole of the scaphoid as a treatment for nonunion. Two patients had to undergo an additional surgical procedure; however, the authors did not find noteworthy wrist collapse. Midcarpal arthritis after distal pole resection did not cause appreciable deterioration in patient outcomes. One important advantage of such a limited and simple surgical approach is that other more extensive salvage procedures can be performed when necessary in the future.

When more advanced scaphoid nonunion advanced collapse wrist deformities are encountered, proximal row carpectomies and partial wrist fusions are more commonly performed. Mulford and colleagues[57] in a systematic review compiled data from 52 articles published from 1980 to 2008 comparing PRC and 4-corner fusion (4CF). The review suggests that grip strength, pain relief, and subjective outcomes are comparable for both surgical groups. Range of motion is also similar in both groups, although it may be slightly less after 4CF. PRC has a higher rate of osteoarthritic change after surgery but 4CF has more complications overall owing to nonunion, dorsal impingement, and complications related to hardware.

Saltzman and colleagues[58] in a meta-analysis reviewed the results of 7 studies comparing PRC and 4CF after all the exclusion criteria were met. The authors found better radial deviation and grip strength in the 4CF group and better flexion, extension, and ulnar deviation, yet a lower complication rate in the PRC group.

We have a preference for PRC over 4CF when the indications overlap. Evidence suggests that even the capitate–radius arthritis seen in long-term outcomes after PRC does not reflect impaired outcomes.[59] In younger high-demand patients or those with lunate–capitate joint arthritis, 4CF, and scaphoid–triquetrum excision and limited lunate–capitate fusion can be performed.[60,61] (**Fig. 4**).

SUMMARY

Surgical strategies for scaphoid nonunions often become more complex based on the time from injury to treatment whereby subsequent development of predictable progressive arthritic processes and adaptive carpal instability occur. The decision-making process, however, can follow a logical sequence as determined by the case grade at presentation. Scaphoid nonunions with less than 1 year after trauma and no carpal malalignment (Slade grades I–III) can be treated with percutaneous screw fixation under either fluoroscopic and/or arthroscopic guidance. We do not see any advantages of the arthroscopy over fluoroscopy with this method. Patients with good proximal poles capable of good screw purchase are good candidates for cortico-cancellous bone grafts. Our preference is structural bone grafts from the iliac crest. Reinterventions or patients with avascular proximal poles that do not need substantial grafts are reliably treated with pedicle vascularized bone grafts. We have a preference for fixation with small (1.5–2.0 mm) screws. In the rare circumstances of significant bone loss and compromised scaphoid proximal poles, free vascularized bone grafts may be indicated and our preference is for the free medial femoral condyle graft. Resection of the distal pole of the scaphoid is a good option in old (>5 years old) or after failed scaphoid procedure in selected patients. When there is radioscaphoid degenerative changes, salvage procedures like PRC or partial wrist fusions (scaphoid and triquetrum excision and lunate–capitate fusion or 4CF) should be considered. Our preference is for PRC unless contraindicated because the technique is simpler, immobilization periods shorter, complications fewer, and outcomes similar to if not superior to more complex interventions.

REFERENCES

1. Breitenseher MJ, Metz VM, Gilula LA. Radiographically occult scaphoid fractures: value of MR imaging in detection. Radiology 1997;203:245–50.
2. Buijze GA, Ochtman L, Ring D. Management of scaphoid nonunion. J Hand Surg Am 2012;37(5): 1095–100.
3. Dias J, Brenkel I, Finlay D. Patterns of union in fractures of the waist of the scaphoid. J Bone Joint Surg Br 1989;71(2):307–10.
4. Merrell GA, Wolfe SW, Slade JF III. Treatment of scaphoid nonunions: quantitative meta-analysis of the literature. J Hand Surg Am 2002;27(4):685–91.
5. Gelberman RH, Menon J. The vascularity of the scaphoid bone. J Hand Surg Am 1980;5(5):508–13.
6. Garcia-Elias M. Understanding wrist mechanics: a long and winding road. J Wrist Surg 2013;2(1):5–12.
7. Kawamura K, Chung KC. Treatment of scaphoid fractures and nonunions. J Hand Surg Am 2008; 33(6):988–97.
8. Schuind F, Haentjens P, Van Innis F, et al. Prognostic factors in the treatment of carpal scaphoid nonunions. J Hand Surg Am 1999;24(4):761–7.
9. Slade JF III, Dodds SD. Minimally invasive management of scaphoid nonunions. Clin Orthop Relat Res 2006;445:108–19.
10. Slade JF III, Geissler WB, Gutow AP, et al. Percutaneous internal fixation of selected scaphoid non-unions with an arthroscopically assisted dorsal approach. J Bone Joint Surg Am 2003;85(Suppl 4):20–32.
11. Slade JF 3rd, Gillon T. Retrospective review of 234 scaphoid fractures and nonunions treated with arthroscopy for union and complications. Scand J Surg 2008;97(4):280–9.
12. Capo JT, Shamian B, Rizzo M. Percutaneous screw fixation without bone grafting of scaphoid non-union. Isr Med Assoc J 2012; 14(12):729–32.
13. Kim JK, Kim JO, Lee SY. Volar percutaneous screw fixation for scaphoid waist delayed union. Clin Orthop Relat Res 2010;468(4):1066–71.
14. Somerson JS, Fletcher DJ, Srinivasan RC, et al. Compression screw fixation without bone grafting for scaphoid fibrous nonunion. Hand (N Y) 2015; 10(3):450–3.
15. Vanhees M, Van Riet RRP, Van Haver A, et al. Percutaneous, transtrapezial fixation without bone graft leads to consolidation in selected cases of delayed union of the scaphoid waist. J Wrist Surg 2017;6(3): 183–7.
16. Hegazy G. Percutaneous screw fixation of scaphoid waist fracture non-union without bone grafting. J Hand Microsurg 2015;7(2):250–5.
17. Mahmoud M, Koptan W. Percutaneous screw fixation without bone grafting for established scaphoid nonunion with substantial bone loss. J Bone Joint Surg Br 2011;93(7):932–6.
18. Cooney WP, Linscheid RL, Dobyns JH, et al. Scaphoid non union: role of anterior interpositional grafts. J Hand Surg 1988;13A:635–50.
19. Fernandez DL. A technique for anterior wedge shaped grafts for scaphoid non unions with carpal instability. J Hand Surg 1984;9A:733–7.
20. Green DP. The effect of avascular necrosis on Russe bone grafting for scaphoid non-union. J Hand Surg 1985;10A:597–605.
21. Watson HK, Pitts EC, Ashmead D, et al. Dorsal approach to scaphoid nonunion. J Hand Surg 1993;18A:359–65.
22. Tambe AD, Cutler L, Murali SR, et al. In scaphoid non-union, does the source of graft affect out-come? Iliac crest versus distal end of radius bone graft. J Hand Surg Br 2006; 31(1):47–51.
23. Garg B, Goyal T, Kotwal PP, et al. Local distal radius bone graft versus iliac crest bone graft for scaphoid nonunion: a comparative study. Musculoskelet Surg 2013;97(2):109–14.
24. Kim JK, Yoon JO, Baek H. Corticocancellous bone graft vs cancellous bone graft for the management of unstable scaphoid nonunion. Orthop Traumatol Surg Res 2018;104(1):115–20.

25. Sayegh ET, Strauch RJ. Graft choice in the management of unstable scaphoid nonunion: a systematic review. J Hand Surg Am 2014;39(8):1500–6.e7.

26. Roy-Camille R. Fractures et pseudarthroses du scaphoïde carpien. Utilisation d'un greffon pédiculé. *Acta Chir Orthop* 1965;4:197–214.

27. Kawai H, Yamamoto K. Pronator quadratus pedicled bone graft for old scaphoid fractures. J Bone Joint Surg Br 1988;70(5):829–31.

28. Kuhlmann JN, Mimoun M, Boabighi A, et al. Vascularized bone graft pedicled on the volar carpal artery for non-union of the scaphoid. J Hand Surg Br 1987;12(2):203–10.

29. Mathoulin C, Haerle M. Vascularized bone graft from the palmar carpal artery for treatment of scaphoid nonunion. J Hand Surg Br 1998;23(3):318–23.

30. Zaidemberg C, Siebert JW, Angrigiani C. A new vascularized bone graft for scaphoid nonunion. J Hand Surg Am 1991;16(3):474–8.

31. Sheetz KK, Bishop AT, Berger RA. The arterial blood supply of the distal radius and ulna and its potential use in vascularized pedicled bone grafts. J Hand Surg 1995;20A:902–14.

32. Guimberteau JC, Panconi B. Recalcitrant non-union of the scaphoid treated with a vascularized bone graft based on the ulnar artery. J Bone Joint Surg Am 1990;72(1):88–97.

33. Bertelli JA, Tacca CP, Rost JR. Thumb metacarpal vascularized bone graft in long-standing scaphoid nonunion-a useful graft via dorsal or palmar approach: a cohort study of 24 patients. J Hand Surg Am 2004;29(6):1089–97.

34. Sotereanos DG, Darlis NA, Dailiana ZH, et al. A capsular-based vascularized distal radius graft for proximal pole scaphoid pseudarthrosis. J Hand Surg Am 2006;31(4):580–7.

35. Antoniou IK, Athanaselis ED, Rountas C, et al. MR angiogram confirms sustained blood flow in 1,2 ICSR artery of vascularized bone grafting in scaphoid nonunion treatment. Eur J Orthop Surg Traumatol 2019;29(2):343–8.

36. Ribak S, Medina CE, Mattar R Jr, et al. Treatment of scaphoid nonunion with vascularised and nonvascularised dorsal bone grafting from the distal radius. Int Orthop 2010;34(5):683–8.

37. Caporrino FA, Dos Santos JB, Penteado FT, et al. Dorsal vascularized grafting for scaphoid nonunion: a comparison of two surgical techniques. J Orthop Trauma 2014;28(3):e44–8.

38. Pinder RM, Brkljac M, Rix L, et al. Treatment of scaphoid nonunion: a systematic review of the existing evidence. J Hand Surg Am 2015;40(9):1797–805.

39. Alluri RK, Yin C, Iorio ML, et al. A critical appraisal of vascularized bone grafting for scaphoid nonunion. J Wrist Surg 2017;6(3):251–7.

40. Gunal I, Ozcelik A, Gokturk E, et al. Correlation of magnetic resonance imaging and intraoperative punctate bleeding to assess the vascularity of scaphoid nonunion. Arch Orthop Trauma Surg 1999;119:285–7.

41. Bervian MR, Ribak S, Livani B. Scaphoid fracture nonunion: correlation of radiographic imaging, proximal fragment histologic viability evaluation, and estimation of viability at surgery. Int Orthop 2015;39:67–72.

42. Donati O, Zanetti M, Nagy L, et al. Is dynamic gadolinium enhancement needed in MR imaging for the preoperative assessment of scaphoidal viability in patients with scaphoid nonunion? Radiology 2011;260:808–16.

43. Kim J, Park JW, Chung J, et al. Non-vascularized iliac bone grafting for scaphoid nonunion with avascular necrosis. J Hand Surg Eur Vol 2018;43(1):24–31.

44. Putnan JG, DiGiovanni RM, Mitchell SM. Plate fixation with cancellous graft for scaphoid nonunion with avascular necrosis. J Hand Surg Am 2019;44(4):339.e1-e7.

45. Chang MA, Bishop AT, Moran SL, et al. The outcomes and complications of 1,2-intercompartmental supraretinacular artery pedicled vascularized bone grafting of scaphoid nonunions. J Hand Surg Am 2006;31(3):387–96.

46. Ferguson DO, Shanbhag V, Hedley H, et al. Scaphoid fracture non-union: a systematic review of surgical treatment using bone graft. J Hand Surg Eur Vol 2016;41(5):492–500.

47. Doi K, Oda T, Soo-Heong T, et al. Free vascularized bone graft for nonunion of the scaphoid. J Hand Surg Am 2000;25(3):507–19.

48. Jones DB Jr, Moran SL, Bishop AT, et al. Free-vascularized medial femoral condyle bone transfer in the treatment of scaphoid nonunions. Plast Reconstr Surg 2010;125(4):1176–84.

49. Al-Jabri T, Mannan A, Giannoudis P. The use of the free vascularised bone graft for nonunion of the scaphoid: a systematic review. J Orthop Surg Res 2014;9:21.

50. Elgammal A, Lukas B. Vascularized medial femoral condyle graft for management of scaphoid nonunion. J Hand Surg Eur Vol 2015;40(8):848–54.

51. Jones DB Jr, Bürger H, Bishop AT, et al. Treatment of scaphoid waist nonunions with an avascular proximal pole and carpal collapse. A comparison of two vascularized bone grafts. J Bone Joint Surg Am 2008;90(12):2616–25.

52. Aibinder WR, Wagner ER, Bishop AT, et al. Bone grafting for scaphoid nonunions: is free vascularized bone grafting superior for scaphoid nonunion? Hand (N Y) 2019;14(2):217–22.

53. Windhofer C, Wong VW, Larcher L, et al. Knee donor site morbidity following harvest of

medial femoral trochlea osteochondral flaps for carpal reconstruction. J Hand Surg Am 2016;41(5): 610–4.e1.

54. Trumble TE, Salas P, Barthel T, et al. Management of scaphoid nonunions. J Am Acad Orthop Surg 2003;11(6):380–91.

55. Milone MT, Klifto CS, Catalano LW III. Partial wrist denervation: the evidence behind a small fix for big problems. J Hand Surg Am 2018; 43(03):272–7.

56. Malerich MM, Catalano LW 3rd, Weidner ZD, et al. Distal scaphoid resection for degenerative arthritis secondary to scaphoid nonunion: a 20-year experience. J Hand Surg Am 2014;39(9): 1669–76.

57. Mulford JS, Ceulemans LJ, Nam D, et al. Proximal row carpectomy VS four corner fusion for scapholunate (SLAC) or scaphoid nonunion advanced

collapse (SNAC) wrists: a systematic review of outcomes. J Hand Surg Eur Vol 2009;34E(2):256–63.

58. Saltzman BM, Frank JM, Slikker W, et al. Clinical outcomes of proximal row carpectomy versus four-corner arthrodesis for post-traumatic wrist arthropathy: a systematic review. J Hand Surg Eur Vol 2015;40(5):450–7.

59. Jebson PJL, Hayes EP, Engber WD. Proximal row carpectomy: a minimum 10-year follow-up study. J Hand Surg 2003;28A:561–9.

60. Calandruccio JH, Gelberman RH, Duncan SF, et al. Capitolunate arthrodesis with scaphoid and triquetrum excision. J Hand Surg 2000;25:824–32.

61. Gaston RG, Greenberg JA, Baltera RM, et al. Clinical outcomes of scaphoid and triquetral excision with capitolunate arthrodesis versus scaphoid excision and four-corner arthrodesis. J Hand Surg 2009; 34:1407–12.

Current Techniques in Scapholunate Ligament Reconstruction

Ian Mullikin, MD[a],*, Ramesh C. Srinivasan, MD[b,c],
Mark Bagg, MD[b]

KEYWORDS

- Scapholunate ligament • Repair • Reconstruction • Salvage • Treatment

KEY POINTS

- Perioperative counseling is paramount in patients with scapholunate ligament injury without evidence of arthrosis.
- Surgeons should approach patients with a treatment algorithm regarding ability to repair and or reconstruct the scapholunate ligament depending on reducibility of the deformity and absence of degenerative arthritis.
- Many repair and reconstructive techniques exist for scapholunate ligament reconstruction with no single, clear advantageous technique.
- Salvage operations exist when repair or reconstruction is not possible; however, nonoperative treatment modalities are sufficient in some individuals.

INTRODUCTION

Scapholunate (SL) ligament injury is a common injury to the wrist and often the result of a high-energy mechanism or fall. Often these injuries are missed and untreated during the acute phase when direct repair of the ligament is possible. Surgeons are often left to choose from a myriad of reconstructive techniques designed to reproduce the best carpal kinematics while attempting to restore strength and range of motion (ROM) of the wrist. It is well established that, if left untreated there is a staged pattern of predictable arthritis that develops in the carpus.[1] Therefore, treatment of these injuries before the development of arthritis is critical. This article outlines the reconstructive options that are available.

ANATOMY AND BIOMECHANICS

The SL ligament is a C-shaped ligament that is composed of 3 main segments: a dorsal, proximal,

and palmar segment.[2] The dorsal region of the ligament is the thickest component and is composed of transversely oriented collagen fibers that contribute most of the ligament's tensile strength.[2,3] This dorsal segment primarily controls flexion and extension and contributes up to 300 N of tensile strength to the ligament complex.[4] In contrast, the proximal portion of the ligament is composed primarily of fibrocartilage with a few longitudinally oriented collagen fibrils. This section of the ligament is considered the weakest portion of the ligament, contributing only 25 to 50 N of tensile strength to the ligament complex.[4] The proximal and palmar segments of the ligament are separated by the radioscapholunate ligament. Last, the palmar section of the ligament is composed primarily of obliquely oriented collagen fibrils that lie just dorsal to the long radiolunate ligament.[2] This volar section of the ligament is largely responsible for controlling rotational motion.[4]

There are also several other secondary stabilizers of the SL ligament complex, such

[a] Department of Orthopedics, 1 Jarrett White Road, Tripler Army Medical Center, HI 96859, USA; [b] Hand Center of San Antonio, 21 Spurs Lane Suite #310, San Antonio, TX 78240, USA; [c] Department of Orthopaedic Surgery, UT San Antonio, San Antonio, TX, USA
* Corresponding author.
E-mail address: ianmullikin@gmail.com

Orthop Clin N Am 51 (2020) 77–86
https://doi.org/10.1016/j.ocl.2019.09.002
0030-5898/20/Published by Elsevier Inc.

as the radioscaphocapitate ligament and scaphotrapezial-trapezoid (STT) ligaments. Sectioning of these ligaments has shown the SL ligament to be the primary stabilizer; however, these ligaments have shown important stabilizing characteristics at the extremes of wrist motion.[5–7] The dart-throwing motion has been proposed as an oblique plane of motion in which the wrist moves from radial extension to ulnar flexion and, in this manner, motion is minimized through the SL joint. This concept has been adapted to initiate early functional rehabilitation without placing undue strain on the ligamentous repair or reconstruction.[8]

CLASSIFICATION

Garcia-Elias and colleagues[9] proposed 5 important prognostic factors to consider when evaluating SL ligament injuries:

1. Is the dorsal SL ligament intact?
2. If the dorsal SL ligament is disrupted, can it be repaired with good healing potential?
3. Is the scaphoid aligned normally with an radioscaphoid angle of 45° or less, indicating a normal STT capsule and ligaments?
4. Is the carpal malalignment easily reducible?
5. Is the cartilage at both radiocarpal and midcarpal joints normal?

They proposed that, by answering these questions, each case could be subdivided into one of 6 different stages, with an associated treatment algorithm for each group. The various stages are detailed as follows[9]:

1. Partial SL ligament injury
2. Complete SL ligament injury with repairable ligament
3. Complete nonrepairable SL ligament injury with normally aligned scaphoid
4. Complete SL ligament injury with a nonrepairable reducible rotary subluxation of the scaphoid
5. Complete SL ligament injury with irreducible malalignment but normal cartilage
6. Complete SL ligament injury with irreducible malalignment and cartilage degeneration

For stages 3 and 4, there is a nonrepairable ligament, with either a normally aligned scaphoid or reducible deformity. In this setting, SL ligament reconstruction may be considered, and this is the focus of this article.

TREATMENT OPTIONS
Acute Injury with Repairable Ligament
These injuries are usually represented as occurring within 2 to 3 weeks of the inciting traumatic

event. If surgery is attempted during this time interval, direct repair of the ligament is usually possible.[10] The SL ligament almost invariably avulses off the scaphoid and repair techniques focus on using suture anchors with attached sutures to reattach the avulsed ligament. This direct repair is often augmented with a variety of other techniques. A popular treatment method has been to combine direct repair with a capsulodesis procedure. This method was initially described by Lavernia and colleagues,[11] in which horizontal mattress sutures are placed in the avulsed SL ligament, a trough is made on the proximal aspect of the scaphoid, and drill holes are used to reapproximate the ligament back down to the bone, then a capsulodesis is performed. Long-term follow-up of direct repair alone in a study by Minami and colleagues[12] found deterioration of clinical outcomes and increase in SL angle from 50° to 60°, prompting the need for augmentation of the repair with capsulodesis. The capsulodesis was first popularized by Blatt,[13] in which the dorsal capsule is tethered to the scaphoid to prevent aberrant flexion of the scaphoid. In this procedure a 1-cm flap of dorsal capsule and dorsal radiocarpal ligament based off the radius is rotated and anchored to the distal pole of the scaphoid distal to the axis of rotation, approximately 3 to 4 mm proximal to the STT joint. However, this tether across the joint does result in an overall decrease in ROM of the wrist.[13] A modification of this method, known as the Mayo capsulodesis, attempts to correct this by using a portion of the distal intercarpal ligament to tether the scaphoid.[14] Fibers of the dorsal intercarpal ligament insert on the scaphoid ridge and trapezoid but none attach at the distal scaphoid. In this modification, a 5-mm strip of dorsal intercarpal ligament that attaches to the trapezoid is raised, stretched, rotated, and anchored into the distal scaphoid.[14] Biomechanical studies have shown better radiographic outcomes regarding SL angle and gap using the Mayo capsulodesis as opposed to Blatt's[13] initial description.[14] It is critical that the SL angle be easily reducible with joystick k-wires. It is our recommendation that the SL interval be easily reduced with .045 Kirschner wires (K-wires); if it is not easily reducible, this may indicate that the injury is chronic and may be prone to failure. This is a key point in the surgeons' decision-making algorithm. Absent reducibility implies proceeding to either salvage or other temporizing measures. Long-term 8-year follow-up studies of capsulodesis procedures indicate varied outcome measures with an average DASH (disabilities of the arm, shoulder, and hand) score of 28, average grip strength of 38 kg, an 88° arc of motion through flexion and extension with 38° total motion in radial and ulnar deviation, average SL angle of 70°, and SL gap of 2.8 mm. No major complications were noted; however, 8 of 59 patients underwent salvage procedures and 78% had radiographic evidence of progression of arthritis.[15]

Often after direct repair is performed K-wire fixation is performed to stabilize the carpal bones following repair. These pins are classically left in place for 8 to 12 weeks to allow ligamentous healing. Recently, attention has been paid to using temporary screw fixation following direct repair. The SL intercarpal screw (SLIC; Acumed LLC), allows some intercarpal motion but limits the SL gap during healing. This screw is often removed 6 to 9 months after placement. A study by Larson and colleagues[16] showed that, in short-term follow-up, patients augmented with screw fixation had a smaller SL gap compared with K-wire fixation (3.1 mm vs 1.3 mm) and at final follow-up both SL gap and angle were better radiographically compared with the K-wire group. Long-term follow-up studies indicated that patients had overall improvement with mild pain and average flexion-extension arc from 106° and 41° arc of radial and ulnar deviation. The average SL angle was 65° with an SL gap of 2.5 mm. Avascular necrosis (AVN) of the proximal scaphoid was noted in 1 patient; however, the patient was asymptomatic at 7-year follow-up and secondary surgery was required for screw removal in all patients at an average of 5 months postoperatively.[17]

Subacute/Chronic Injuries Without Repairable Ligament: Reducible Deformity

In settings in which the injury presents outside of the acute period, which is classically regarded as the first 3 months from injury, a myriad of interventions have been championed. A variety of tendon weave procedures, screw fixation, bone-ligament-bone systems, and new implant devices have been proposed. In the case of a subacute chronic injury with a normally aligned scaphoid, one option is to perform a bone-ligament-bone graft as proposed by Weiss.[18] This initial description used a graft from the dorsal distal radius with variable results, and later other graft options were described. A popular option is now the metacarpal-carpal grafts described by Harvey and colleagues.[19] Grafts from the base of either the third or second metacarpal correlate to the strength and stiffness of

the native SL ligament.[19] Morrell and Weiss[20] reported on long-term follow-up bone-retinaculum-bone autografts over an average of 11.9 years. Overall Mayo wrist score was 83, with an average grip strength of 38 kg. The overall flexion-extension arc was 97° with a 65° SL angle and 3.5 mm SL gap. Various complications were noted, including neuroma of the radial sensory nerve and breakdown over the fixation pin. Three patients (21%) required revision to either proximal row carpectomy (PRC) or arthrodesis.[20]

There have also been several differing tendon weaves proposed, designed to tether motion across the scaphoid. This method was first brought to the forefront by Brunelli and Brunelli.[21] A 7-cm strip of flexor carpi radialis (FCR) is harvested, maintaining its attachment to the base of the second metacarpal, and the slip is then passed through a 2.5-mm drill tunnel running from a volar to dorsal direction through the axis of the scaphoid. This tendon slip is then sutured to the dorsal distal radius and fibrous remains of the lunate.[21] This technique has subsequently been altered by Van Den Abbeele[22] to avoid crossing the radiocarpal joint.

A slightly different tendon weave modification was devised by Almquist and colleagues[23] in which a strip of the extensor carpi radialis brevis (ECRB) is harvested and woven through drill tunnels placed in the scaphoid, lunate, capitate, and distal radius. The tendon is first passed in a dorsal to volar direction through the capitate before being brought back out dorsally through the lunate. The graft is then brought palmarly through the scaphoid before being brought back out dorsally through the distal radius and sutured into the periosteum.[23]

Another modification of the Brunelli technique is the triligament tenodesis technique. The FCR tendon is woven through the axis of the scaphoid, which is then used to recreate the dorsal radial triquetral ligament, scaphotrapeziotrapezoid, and SL ligaments.[9]

Long-term follow-up of the Brunelli weave and various modifications showed that only 1 of 8 patients went on to develop radiographic arthritis, and complex regional pain syndrome was noted as a possible complication; however, there was evidence of loss of reduction at final follow-up. Loss of the SL angle and gap was observed over the 10-year follow-up period, with an overall SL gap of 2.4 mm and 63° SL angle. Clinically, 6 of the 8 patients reported a pain-free wrist with an average DASH score of 9. Grip strength was 85% of the contralateral side and the overall flexion-extension arc was also 85% of the contralateral wrist.[24]

The RASL (reduction and association of the scaphoid and the lunate) procedure creates an intentional fibrous nonunion between the scaphoid and the lunate using a compression screw across the axis of the scaphoid to make a neoligament, allowing motion.[25] A recent functional and radiographic outcome study on the RASL technique showed that pain scores unanimously improved; however, ROM and grip strength decreased. In addition, progressive arthritis was observed in more than 50% of the patients and symptomatic hardware loosening required screw removal in several of the patients.[26] In a follow-up study by Larson and Stern,[27] overall patient outcomes showed an average DASH score of 15, with grip strength of 77% of the contralateral wrist and a flexion-extension arc of 99°. Radiographically the SL angle was 59° with a 4.5-mm SL gap. However, during the study 5 of 8 patients were noticed to develop arthritic changes. As a result, the investigators recommended abandoning the procedure.[27] Recently, Koehler and colleagues[28] showed that accurate placement of the RASL screw proximal to the lateral aspect of the scaphoid dorsal ridge was crucial for maximizing biomechanical stability and associated clinical outcome. Perhaps the results reported by these other studies would be improved with optimal screw placement.

Alternatively, the SL ligament can be reconstructed using a palmaris longus tendon graft using 2 suture anchors, without passing the tendon graft through drill holes in the scaphoid and lunate. Four-year follow-up data of this technique showed that most patients were able to return to work and were satisfied with their procedures, with an average DASH score of 29% and 75% of grip strength and ROM compared with the contralateral hand.[29] A modification of this procedure has been devised using the Arthrex Internal Brace, which has been gaining in popularity recently. Although only 1 case report is currently published, their 13-month follow-up showed that the patient had returned to work with normal carpal alignment.[30]

Recently, there have been attempts to recreate both the volar and dorsal aspects of the SL ligament. The SL axis method (SLAM) technique creates a multiplanar connection between the scaphoid and lunate with a tendon graft that is passed through the central axis of the scaphoid and lunate combined with reconstruction of the critical dorsal portion of the ligament. Initial reports were promising: the SLAM technique seemed to be superior to standard capsulodesis and modified Brunelli techniques when tested biomechanically.[31] One-year follow-up showed a reduction in patients' overall pain scores with average grip strength 62% of the contralateral side and a flexion-extension arc of 101°. Radiographic follow-up showed an SL angle of 59° and SL gap of 2.1 mm. However, significant complications have been reported, including 2 cases of AVN of the lunate when using the SLAM technique.[29,30] At our institution, our only case of SLAM reconstruction resulted in AVN of the proximal pole of the scaphoid.

Additional techniques have emerged attempting to recreate both volar and dorsal limbs of the SL ligament to better restore the natural kinematics of the wrist. Henry[32] described harvesting a strip of the FCR and passing it through the scaphoid in a volar to dorsal direction as Brunelli and Brunelli[21] had described, and then passing it from dorsal to volar through the lunate, passing the residual FCR strip back on itself to recreate the volar limb.

Recently, arthroscopic-assisted reduction of the scaphoid and lunate using a palmaris tendon graft in a boxlike reconstruction has been described.[33] Four-year follow-up data showed overall reduction in visual analog scale (VAS) pain scores and grip strength of 84% of the contralateral wrist. The overall flexion-extension arc was 112° with a 51° arc of radial and ulnar deviation. There was no comment on the SL angle; however, SL gap was 2.9 mm on average. AVN of the proximal pole of the scaphoid was noted as well; and 4 out of 17 patients developed residual dorsal intercalated segment instability (DISI) deformity.[33]

Corella and colleagues[34,35] reported a cadaveric model of SL ligament reconstruction that also included volar ligament reconstruction. Short-term (6-month) follow-up showed near full return of ROM and improved grip strength, but no long-term follow-up has been published.[34,35]

Table 1 summarizes the main clinical and radiographic outcomes of each main reconstructive option for SL reconstruction.

When faced with subacute/chronic injuries without arthritic changes and an irreparable ligament, the preference at our institution is to attempt reconstruction using the Arthrex Internal Brace augmented with a slip of the ECRB tendon shown in Fig. 1. In this technique, SwiveLock anchors with the tendon graft are used to secure the central portion of the lunate to the

Table 1
Clinical and radiographic outcomes of scapholunate reconstructive options

Procedure	Patient Outcomes	Grip Strength	Range of Motion	SL°	SL Gap (mm)	Complications	Survivorship/Revision Surgery	Follow-up
Dorsal intercarpal capsulodesis[15]	DASH 28 Mayo 61	38.2 kg	88° (flex/ext arc) 38° (radial-ulnar deviation)	70	2.8	None reported	8 out of 59 underwent salvage procedures, 78% with radiographic arthritis progression	8.25 y
SLIC screw[17]	Good, with mild pain	—	106° (flex/ext arc) 41° (radial-ulnar deviation)	56	2.5	AVN of proximal scaphoid,	Yes; screw removal	7.9 y
BTB[35]	Mayo 83	38 kg	97° (flex/ext arc)	65	3.5	SBRN neuroma, skin breakdown over fixation pin	3 patients requiring revision to prc/arthrodesis	11.9 y
Modified	Mayo 83 DASH 9	85% of contralateral	85% of contralateral wrist	63	2.4	CRPS	1 patient with posttraumatic arthritis	13.8 y
RASL[27]	PRWE 26 DASH 15	77% of contralateral	99° (flex/ext arc)	59	4.5	Screw loosening/removal	5 of 8 patients with failure	3.2 y
SLAM[30]	Pain VAS 1.7	62% of contralateral	101° (flex/ext arc)	59	2.1	AVN of lunate AVN of scaphoid	1 failure out of 13 patients	11 mo
Combined volar and dorsal reconstruction[32]	Pain VAS 1.8	84% of contralateral	112° (flex/ext arc) 51° (radial-ulnar deviation)	—	2.9	AVN of proximal pole of scaphoid	4 patients with recurrence of DISI	4 y

Abbreviations: BTB, bone -tendon-bone; ext, extension; flex, flexion; mo, months; PRC, proximal row carpectomy; PRWE, patient - rated wrist evaluation; SBRN, superficial branch of radial nerve; y, years.

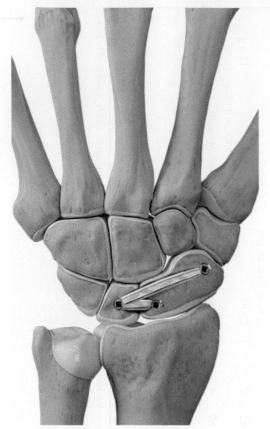

Fig. 1. All-dorsal SL reconstruction with Internal-Brace™ ligament augmentation. (This image was provided courtesy of Arthrex®, Naples, Florida 2019.)

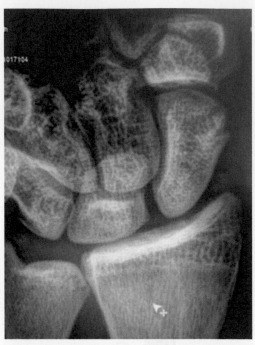

Fig. 2. Radiograph of injury; posteroanterior (PA) view.

dorsal proximal and distal poles of the scaphoid. Figs. 2–4 show hand radiographs of a former National Football League player who presented with a painful SL injury that had not gone on to develop arthritic changes. At last follow-up, 2 years after surgery, he showed excellent wrist ROM, with flexion of 65°, extension of 65° (Figs. 5 and 6), and grip strength of 170 kg on the operative side compared with 160 kg on the uninjured side. At last follow-up he was pain free and had returned to all activities. His 2-year follow-up radiographs are shown in Figs. 7 and 8, with reduction of the SL gap and no progression of arthritic changes.

Irreparable Ligament Injuries and Nonreducible Deformities

In the setting of irreducible deformity with healthy cartilage, different techniques outside of the reconstructive options detailed earlier may be considered. Aggressive mobilization of the scaphoid and lunate may be used in an attempt to convert it to a reducible deformity;

however, the authors caution against such measures. This stage of SL injury is still unsolved in our opinion. In these cases, there should be great consideration of the nonoperative

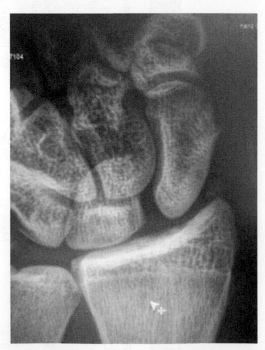

Fig. 3. Radiograph of injury; clenched fist view.

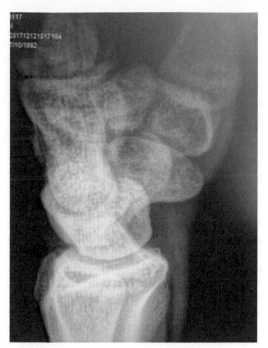

Fig. 4. Radiograph of injury; lateral view.

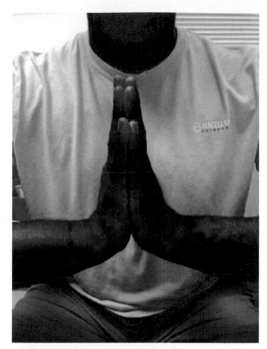

Fig. 6. Extension at final follow-up.

treatment modalities used for SL injury. These treatment modalities include splinting, antiin-flammatories, and steroid injections. There is no methodology described in the literature to help guide surgeons know preoperatively whether or not the deformity will be reducible without opening the wrist and attempting reduc-tion. In such cases, the authors advise a thor-ough preoperative counseling discussion with

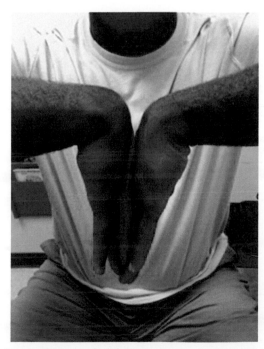

Fig. 5. Flexion at final follow-up.

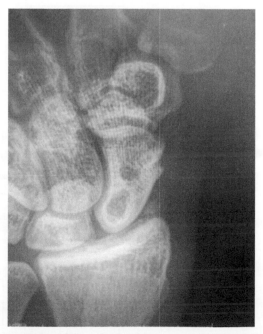

Fig. 7. Final follow-up; PA view.

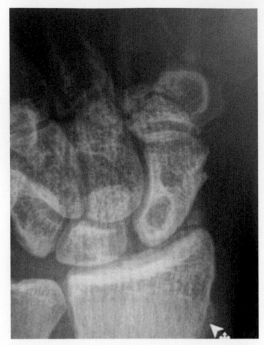

Fig. 8. Final follow-up; clenched fist view.

the patient regarding potential treatment scenarios. In some cases, it may be best to close the wrist and treat conservatively, before

proceeding to more salvage-type operations in patients with irreducible deformity and preserved cartilage; **Fig. 9** shows a complete proposed treatment algorithm of SL ligament injuries. However, there are some limited fusions that may be considered, as opposed to full salvage procedures, such as an STT fusion or an isolated scaphocapitate (SC) fusion.[36,37]

Complete Injury with Irreparable Ligament and Degenerative Cartilage

SL ligament injuries go on to develop a predictable pattern of radiographic arthrosis (scaphoid lunate advanced collapse [SLAC] wrist).[1] Once SLAC changes have developed, reconstructive surgery is unlikely to be successful. Salvage procedures, including proximal row carpectomy, scaphoidectomy with partial wrist fusion such as a 4-corner or central column capitolunate fusion, and total wrist arthrodesis are the most common treatment options. Further discussion of these treatment options is outside the scope of this article. However, it is our preference to perform proximal row carpectomies in the setting of degenerative SLAC wrists that have failed appropriate nonoperative interventions such as antiinflammatories, bracing, and injections.

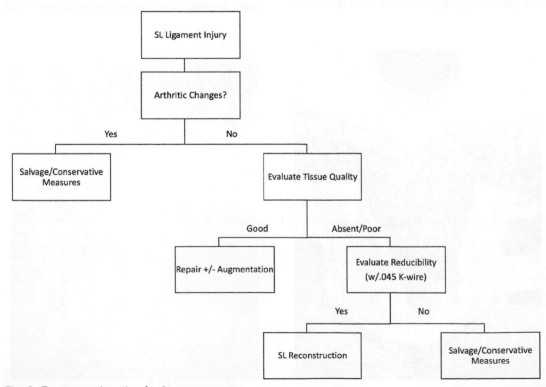

Fig. 9. Treatment algorithm for SL reconstruction.

SUMMARY

Complete SL disruptions can lead to SLAC wrist deformity with associated loss of motion, loss of grip strength, and disability. Early recognition and treatment is ideal. If unrecognized or if patients present late with a chronic injury, various reconstruction options have been described with variable success. Additional prospective randomized control trials are needed comparing these various techniques with longer follow-up intervals to assess the durability of these procedures.

DISCLOSURE

I. Mullikin, R. Srinivasan, M. Bagg: research grant from Acumed. R. Srinivasan: speakers bureau.

REFERENCES

1. Watson HK, Ballet FL. The SLAC wrist: scapholunate advanced collapse pattern of degenerative arthritis. J Hand Surg Am 1984;9(3):358–65.
2. Berger RA. The gross and histologic anatomy of the scapholunate interosseous ligament. J Hand Surg Am 1996;21(2):170–8.
3. Buijze GA, Lozano-Calderon SA, Strackee SD, et al. Osseous and ligamentous scaphoid anatomy: Part I. A systematic literature review highlighting controversies. J Hand Surg Am 2011;36(12):1926–35.
4. Sokolow C, Saffar P. Anatomy and histology of the scapholunate ligament. Hand Clin 2001;17(1):77–81.
5. Short WH, Werner FW, Green JK, et al. Biomechanical evaluation of ligamentous stabilizers of the scaphoid and lunate. J Hand Surg Am 2002;27(6):991–1002.
6. Short WH, Werner FW, Green JK, et al. Biomechanical evaluation of the ligamentous stabilizers of the scaphoid and lunate: Part II. J Hand Surg Am 2005; 30(1):24–34.
7. Short WH, Werner FW, Green JK, et al. Biomechanical evaluation of the ligamentous stabilizers of the scaphoid and lunate: part III. J Hand Surg Am 2007; 32(3):297–309.
8. Crisco JJ, Coburn JC, Moore DC, et al. In vivo radiocarpal kinematics and the dart thrower's motion. J Bone Joint Surg Am 2005;87(12):2729–40.
9. Garcia-Elias M, Lluch AL, Stanley JK. Three-ligament tenodesis for the treatment of scapholunate dissociation: indications and surgical technique. J Hand Surg Am 2006;31(1):125–34.
10. Beredjiklian PK, Dugas J, Gerwin M. Primary repair of the scapholunate ligament. Tech Hand Up Extrem Surg 1998;2(4):269–73.
11. Lavernia CJ, Cohen MS, Taleisnik J. Treatment of scapholunate dissociation by ligamentous repair and capsulodesis. J Hand Surg Am 1992;17(2): 354–9.
12. Minami A, Kato H, Iwasaki N. Treatment of scapholunate dissociation: ligamentous repair associated with modified dorsal capsulodesis. Hand Surg 2003;8(1):1–6.
13. Blatt G. Capsulodesis in reconstructive hand surgery. Dorsal capsulodesis for the unstable scaphoid and volar capsulodesis following excision of the distal ulna. Hand Clin 1987;3(1):81–102.
14. Slater RR, Szabo RM, Bay BK, et al. Dorsal intercarpal ligament capsulodesis for scapholunate dissociation: biomechanical analysis in a cadaver model. J Hand Surg Am 1999;24(2):232–9.
15. Megerle K, Bertel D, Germann G, et al. Long-term results of dorsal intercarpal ligament capsulodesis for the treatment of chronic scapholunate instability. J Bone Joint Surg Br 2012;94(12):1660–5.
16. Larson TB, Gaston RG, Chadderdon RC. The use of temporary screw augmentation for the treatment of scapholunate injuries. Tech Hand Up Extrem Surg 2012;16(3):135–40.
17. Fok MW, Fernandez DL. Chronic scapholunate instability treated with temporary screw fixation. J Hand Surg Am 2015;40(4):752–8.
18. Weiss AP. Scapholunate ligament reconstruction using a bone-retinaculum-bone autograft. J Hand Surg Am 1998;23(2):205–15.
19. Harvey EJ, Berger RA, Osterman AL, et al. Bone-tissue-bone repairs for scapholunate dissociation. J Hand Surg Am 2007;32(2):256–64.
20. Morrell NT, Weiss AP. Bone-retinaculum-bone autografts for scapholunate interosseous ligament reconstruction. Hand Clin 2015;31(3):451–6.
21. Brunelli GA, Brunelli GR. A new technique to correct carpal instability with scaphoid rotary subluxation: a preliminary report. J Hand Surg Am 1995; 20(3 Pt 2):S82–5.
22. Van Den Abbeele KL, Loh YC, Stanley JK, et al. Early results of a modified Brunelli procedure for scapholunate instability. J Hand Surg Br 1998; 23(2):258–61.
23. Almquist EE, Bach AW, Sack JT, et al. Four-bone ligament reconstruction for treatment of chronic complete scapholunate separation. J Hand Surg Am 1991;16(2):322–7.
24. Nienstedt F. Treatment of static scapholunate instability with modified Brunelli tenodesis: results over 10 years. J Hand Surg Am 2013;38(5):887–92.
25. Rosenwasser MP, Miyasajsa KC, Strauch RJ. The RASL procedure: reduction and association of the scaphoid and lunate using the Herbert screw. Tech Hand Up Extrem Surg 1997;1(4):263–72.
26. Aibinder WR, Izadpanah A, Elhassan BT. Reduction and association of the scaphoid and lunate: a functional and radiographical outcome study. J Wrist Surg 2019;8(1):37–42.
27. Larson TB, Stern PJ. Reduction and association of the scaphoid and lunate procedure: short-term

clinical and radiographic outcomes. J Hand Surg Am 2014;39(11):2168–74.

28. Koehler SM, Beck CM, Nasser P, et al. The effect of screw trajectory for the reduction and association of the scaphoid and lunate (RASL) procedure: a biomechanical analysis. J Hand Surg Eur Vol 2018; 43(6):635–41.

29. Gandhi MJ, Knight TP, Ratcliffe PJ. Scapholunate ligament reconstruction using the palmaris longus tendon and suture anchor fixation in chronic scapholunate instability. Indian J Orthop 2016;50(6):616–21.

30. Kakar S, Greene RM. Scapholunate Ligament Internal Brace 360-Degree Tenodesis (SLITT) Procedure. J Wrist Surg 2018;7(4):336–40.

31. Lee SK, Zlotolow DA, Sapienza A, et al. Biomechanical comparison of 3 methods of scapholunate ligament reconstruction. J Hand Surg Am 2014;39(4):643–50.

32. Henry M. Reconstruction of both volar and dorsal limbs of the scapholunate interosseous ligament. J Hand Surg Am 2013;38(8):1625–34.

33. Ho PC, Wong CW, Tse WL. Arthroscopic-assisted combined dorsal and volar scapholunate ligament reconstruction with tendon graft for chronic SL instability. J Wrist Surg 2015;4(4):252–63.

34. Corella F, Del Cerro M, Larrainzar-Garijo R, et al. Arthroscopic ligamentoplasty (bone-tendon-tenodesis). A new surgical technique for scapholunate instability: preliminary cadaver study. J Hand Surg Eur Vol 2011;36(8):682–9.

35. Corella F, Del Cerro M, Ocampos M, et al. Arthroscopic ligamentoplasty of the dorsal and volar portions of the scapholunate ligament. J Hand Surg Am 2013;38(12):2466–77.

36. Watson HK, Ryu J, Akelman E. Limited triscaphoid intercarpal arthrodesis for rotatory subluxation of the scaphoid. J Bone Joint Surg Am 1986;68(3): 345–9.

37. Watson HK, Weinzweig J, Guidera PM, et al. One thousand intercarpal arthrodeses. J Hand Surg Br 1999;24(3):307–15.

Shoulder and Elbow

Proximal Humeral Bone Loss in Revision Shoulder Arthroplasty

Timothy Kahn, MD, Peter N. Chalmers, MD*

KEYWORDS

- Revision shoulder arthroplasty • Proximal humeral bone loss • Allograft prosthesis composite
- Humeral endoprosthesis

KEY POINTS

- It is important to identify and classify the extent of proximal humeral bone loss preoperatively, with a plan to address humeral length, stem fixation issues, and bone stock.
- Causes of proximal humeral bone loss include infection, stress shielding, difficult stem removal, aseptic loosening of previous implant, and osteolysis secondary to wear debris.
- Reconstructive options include a cemented long stem with possible greater tuberosity fixation, an allograft composite prosthesis using proximal humeral or femoral allograft, and proximal/total humeral endoprosthetic replacements.
- It is important to use a monoblock humeral prosthesis in the setting of bone loss to avoid prosthesis failure.

INTRODUCTION

As the number of shoulder arthroplasty procedures performed continues to grow annually,[1] the volume of revision arthroplasty procedures is likely to increase proportionately. Furthermore, as shoulder arthroplasty is increasingly being used for younger patient populations,[2] the burden of revisions can be expected to be even greater.

Revision shoulder arthroplasty is a challenging procedure that has been shown to have inferior outcomes and higher complication rates when compared with primary shoulder arthroplasty.[3–6] However, revision arthroplasty has also been shown to confer substantial benefits to the patient, with several studies demonstrating improvement in function, pain, and range of motion (ROM), even if inferior to primary shoulder arthroplasty outcomes.[7–9]

Of the several reconstructive challenges that face revision shoulder arthroplasty, proximal humeral bone loss is one of the most daunting obstacles to achieving a well-fixed, stable prosthesis.[10,11] Because proximal humeral bone loss compromises proximal bony fixation and potential ingrowth into the humeral stem, the implant relies on rotational stability within the diaphysis. This situation has been shown to increase rotational micromotion, and suggests a higher risk of stem loosening.[11] Described causes of humeral bone loss in the setting of revision arthroplasty include stress shielding, aseptic loosening of the humeral component, osteolysis attributable to wear debris or ongoing infection, previous fracture with subsequent resorption,[10] or bone loss

---

This study did not receive any financial support.

Disclaimer: None.

Disclosures: The authors declare that he has no conflicts of interest in the authorship or publication of this contribution.

Department of Orthopaedic Surgery, University of Utah Medical Center, 590 Wakara Way, Salt Lake City, UT 84108, USA

* Corresponding author.

E-mail address: p.n.chalmers@gmail.com

Orthop Clin N Am 51 (2020) 87–95
https://doi.org/10.1016/j.ocl.2019.08.003

during extraction of a well-fixed stem.[12] The extent of this bone loss can vary widely, which poses unique challenges depending on the amount and location of the bone loss.

CLASSIFICATION

One of the difficulties in devising consistent treatment strategies in the past was the lack of a reliable or validated means of classifying humeral bone loss. As the character and extent of bone loss is variable, establishing a system that more accurately defines the humeral bone loss is crucial toward building consistent treatment algorithms and effective communication across providers.

Several means of classifying bone loss have been proposed. McLendon and colleagues[13] classified bone loss as either less than or greater than 5 cm of bone loss when measuring from the superior aspect of the medial humeral tray to the medial humeral shaft, which for these investigators served as general indications for the use of an allograft prosthesis composite (APC). Similarly, Boileau[4] recommended using 5 cm of humeral bone loss as a cutoff for deciding between "cementoplasty reconstruction" and APC. However, neither of these classification schemes has been validated.

Recently, another classification system was proposed by Chalmers and colleagues,[14] which describes the more nuanced features of humeral bone loss and correlates these features with common treatment strategies. The Proximal Humeral Arthroplasty Revision Osseous inSufficiency (PHAROS) system includes both a basic numeric and more specific alphanumeric system to classify bone loss. It is the only classification system of proximal humeral bone loss that has demonstrated reliability. Overall, the PHAROS classification system demonstrated agreement between raters on 65% of shoulders evaluated (interobserver reliability: κ = 0.545) and between the same rater over a 4-month period on 71% of shoulders (intraobserver reliability: κ = 0.615). The system uses an anteroposterior, Grashey, and lateral-view (axillary or scapular Y) radiograph only and does not require computed tomography or MRI.

PHAROS type 1 describes epiphyseal bone loss, which includes the articular surface, tuberosities, and calcar. This is further subdivided into type 1C, which specifies calcar loss, and type 1G, which specifies loss or malunion of the greater tuberosity (Fig. 1A, B). In the study by Chalmers and colleagues,[14] type 1 constitutes 31% of patients.

PHAROS type 2 describes metadiaphyseal bone loss, which is defined as the bone proximal to the deltoid attachment. Subdivision type 2A refers to cortical thinning of the metadiaphysis greater than 50% of the expected cortical thickness, with this thickness defined based on the noninstrumented portions of the humerus. Type 2B has bone loss of both the metadiaphysis proximal to the deltoid and the epiphysis (Fig. 1C, D).

PHAROS type 3 describes diaphyseal bone loss extending below the deltoid attachment. Type 3A has cortical thinning of diaphysis greater than 50% of the expected cortical thickness (Fig. 1E), whereas type 3B has compromise of most of the diaphysis, along with loss of epiphyseal and metadiaphyseal bone (Fig. 1F).

This classification has been shown to correlate with treatment: the average stem length used was found to increase in each numeric type, from 130 mm for type 1, to 150 mm for type 2, and to 190 mm for type 3. In general, structural bone grafting was used more often in types 2 and 3. Intraoperative tuberosity fixation was most common in types 1 and 2. Proximal or total humeral endoprosthetic replacement was most common in type 3.

PREOPERATIVE PLANNING

Although advanced imaging may be useful in evaluation of both humeral and glenoid bone loss, an adequate preoperative evaluation of humeral bone loss can most often be achieved with radiographs alone.[12,14] Attention should be given to measuring the length of the humeral implant in place because this will provide intraoperative data regarding the length of the proportional cortical window needed to remove a well-fixed implant. The quality of bone suggested from radiographs may also indicate the need for larger reconstructive efforts, and the surgeon should be prepared for a substantially larger bone defect in the setting of very poor bone quality, especially when combined with a well-fixed stem. When planning for either stem position or the length of the allograft in an APC, it may be beneficial to obtain bilateral full-length humeral radiographs to better evaluate humeral length deficits.

Radiographs should be scrutinized for any evidence of humeral loosening. Although isolated humeral loosening is generally rare,[15] it may be more common in revision reverse total shoulder arthroplasty (RTSA) because of compromised metaphysis and tuberosities, possible glenoid polyethylene debris, or possible cement

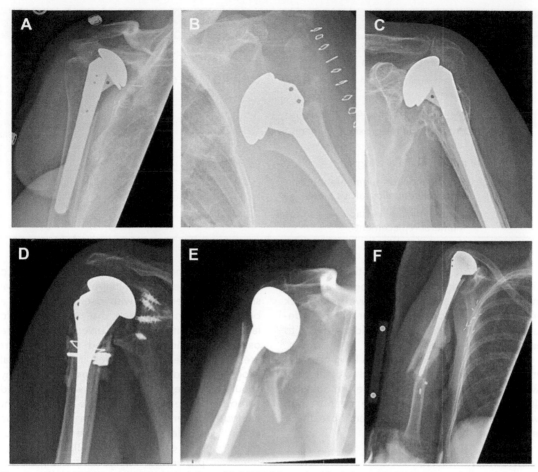

Fig. 1. (A) PHAROS grade 1C bone defect. (B) PHAROS grade 1G defect. (C) PHAROS grade 2A defect. (D) PHAROS grade 2B defect. (E) PHAROS grade 3A defect. (F) PHAROS grade 3B defect.

particles.[12,16] Radiographic signs of loosening include component subsidence, cortical scalloping, radiolucent line formation, and pedestal formation around the distal stem.

In any evaluation of humeral component loosening or osteolysis, it is important to obtain inflammation-related laboratory data (complete blood count, erythrocyte sedimentation rate, C-reactive protein) preoperatively.[17] However, normal laboratory values to do not exclude an infection and if suspicion for infection is high, shoulder aspiration or biopsy should be obtained before surgical planning to rule out infection.

RECONSTRUCTIVE OPTIONS

When addressing proximal humeral bone loss, there are essentially 3 broad categories of treatment strategies to achieve humeral stem fixation. The first is to achieve stem fixation with cement technique alone, restoring length either by cementing the stem proportionately proud or by

using implant modifications as the implant system allows, such as an eccentric glenosphere or thicker polyethylene. The second strategy is to reconstruct the proximal humerus by means of an APC construct. There are several potential means of accomplishing this (see later discussion). The third strategy is that of a proximal humeral or total humeral endoprosthetic replacement.

When deciding on a surgical strategy, both preoperatively and intraoperatively, the PHAROS classification system can help to suggest a basic treatment algorithm (Table 1). Although certainly not comprehensive, this would serve as a framework for surgical planning. For type 1C and type 1G defects, it can be expected that stem fixation will be achieved through cement augmentation alone, leaving the stem proportionately proud to re-establish height. For type 1G defects, special care must be given to restoring anatomic tuberosity positioning and achieving excellent fixation of the tuberosities.[14]

Table 1
Treatment algorithm for proximal humeral bone loss using PHAROS classification

Type/Subtype	Treatment Algorithm	Stem Length (mm)	
1C	Cement augmentation to re-establish height	110–130	Consider bilateral full-length humeral radiographs to assess for humeral length deficits
1G	Evaluate for malreduced tuberosity		
2A	Consideration for proximal humeral allograft	150–170	
2B	Proximal humeral allograft		
3A	Consideration for augmentation with femoral strut allograft vs plate	≥200	
3B	Proximal humeral replacement or total humeral replacement		

For type 2A defects, consideration should be given to a proximal humeral allograft pending the quality and nature of the native bone stock encountered intraoperatively. For type 2B defects, more definitive plans should be made to use a proximal humeral allograft.

Type 3A defects may require a long proximal humerus allograft versus a femoral strut allograft (which can extend up through the metadiaphysis). Type 3B bone defects are best treated with proximal or total humeral endoprosthetic replacement.

APPROACH

Although the location of the skin incision may be partly dictated by previous surgical scars, the authors generally use a standard deltopectoral approach for all revisions. Tissue planes can be difficult to distinguish in the revision setting. The dissection should generally follow the "scar plane," erring medially to avoid damage to the anterior deltoid, and using the palpable coracoid as a secondary guide.[12]

It is important to avoid damaging or deinnervating the anterior deltoid musculature by straying laterally during the deltopectoral dissection. Once the deltoid has been freed from the underlying rotator cuff and humerus, it is possible to re-establish the normal gliding planes of the shoulder, including the subacromial, subdeltoid, and subconjoint spaces.[12] At this point, it is possible to better identify the state of the rotator cuff and whether there is preserved posterior cuff or subscapularis.

HUMERAL COMPONENT REMOVAL

In the revision setting, if the humeral stem is well fixed within the native bone, the removal can be both challenging and potentially destructive to the native bone stock. Initial efforts at removal should be attempted with osteotomes and a burr, attempting to keep the cement mantle largely intact if present. Curved and flexible osteotomes and a high-speed router-tip burr are also very helpful. However, if no substantial progress is made, a vertical humeral osteotomy should be made using a saw followed by stacked osteotomes to better remove the implant without further damaging the native bone stock.[18] Consideration can also be given to a humeral window osteotomy (**Fig. 2**). The authors generally prefer the latter because it provides a better view for the removal of cement with weak bone. Although a vertical humeral osteotomy can be fixed with cerclages, a window osteotomy usually requires matched drill holes so that the osteotomy can be "sewn" back to the humerus.

After the humeral component is removed, a final evaluation of the humeral bone stock should be made. Based on the extent of bone loss, a decision can be made as to which reconstructive option is most suitable to address the defect.

RECONSTRUCTION OPTIONS
Modular Stem Retention

Some newer humeral components have been designed to have a modular humeral stem that can be converted to reverse shoulder arthroplasty without removing the stem. Although this may be an attractive option in a well-fixed stem, one must bear in mind that difficulties can arise with such a system. If the length is inappropriate, version is incorrect, or there is substantial bone loss around the modular junction, removal of the stem may still be necessary.

A   B

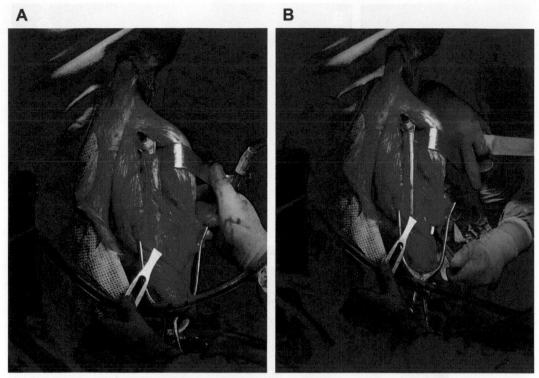

Fig. 2. (A) Demonstration of a well-fixed stem that (B) required a cortical window osteotomy for stem removal.

Furthermore, there is concern for the durability of these modular components in a proximal bone loss setting because the rotational stresses on a reverse stem are substantially different from the rotational stresses on an anatomic stem.[11,19]

In a biomechanical study by Cuff and colleagues,[11] humeral bone loss models were created using Sawbones, and 3 types of stems were implanted into the models (2 modular and 1 monoblock). After 1,000 torsion cycles, all failed constructs, both in bone loss and intact models, were modular rather than monoblock. The investigators concluded that modular implants may be at increased risk of mechanical failure in the setting of proximal humeral bone loss. Based on these findings, as well as several clinical reports of failed modular components, consideration should be given to using monoblock implants for reconstruction constructs in the setting of significant proximal humeral bone loss.

Cemented Arthroplasty Without Allograft
For bone defects isolated to the epiphysis, or some type 2A defects with adequate metadiaphyseal bone stock, a cemented revision without use of an allograft is a reasonable option (Fig. 3A). In the setting of a revision arthroplasty

with previous cementation of the humeral component, cementing into an intact cement mantle is preferable.[19] If a vertical osteotomy was performed for stem removal, this should be repaired using a minimum of 3 cerclage wires secured with a trial implant in place, being careful to protect the radial nerve during passage around the humerus distally.[12]

Because judgment of stem height is crucial toward stability in this setting, it is useful to obtain bilateral full-length humerus radiographs for comparison with the contralateral side. Intraoperatively, adequate length can be determined through use of a trial component before cementation, by evaluating soft tissue/axillary nerve tension, force required to inferiorly subluxate the humerus, and force required for prosthetic dislocation.[12]

Restoring humeral length can be achieved in several ways. Perhaps the most conceptually simple technique is to cement the humeral stem in a proud position that has been determined through preoperative planning and trialing. However, depending on the implant system, there are various means of restoring and modifying the functional length of the humerus, which include metal augmentation at the stem-bone interface or a thicker polyethylene tray. Furthermore, using

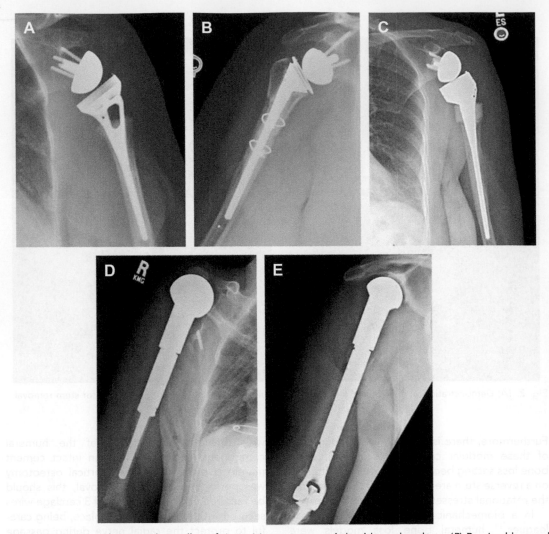

Fig. 3. (A) Cemented stem without allograft in revision reverse total shoulder arthroplasty. (B) Proximal humeral allograft composite prosthesis. (C) Femoral allograft composite prosthesis. (D) Proximal humeral replacement. (E) Total humeral replacement.

a larger glenosphere or an inferiorly eccentric glenosphere can modulate the stability and soft-tissue tension at the joint, compensating for small deficits in humeral length.

Humeral revision using a cemented long-stem monoblock prosthesis without the use of an allograft may be a viable option in the setting of limited metadiaphyseal bone loss.[8,19] The proposed argument for this strategy is that a long-stem humeral component in the setting of the semiconstrained nature of an RTSA prosthesis lends adequate stability without the added risks and costs of a bulk allograft. Budge and colleagues[19] reported a mean improvement in American Shoulder and Elbow Surgeons (ASES) scores for 15 patients with an average bone loss of 38.4 mm who underwent revision RTSA

without allograft augmentation; however, the average follow-up period was less than 3 years and there was an overall complication rate of 47%. Similarly, Stephens and colleagues[8] performed revision RTSA without allograft augmentation on 16 patients with an average proximal humeral bone loss of 36.3 mm. Likewise, there was a mean improvement in ASES scores at final follow-up (average of 51.2 months), but the overall complication rate was 31%, and 3 of the patients developed humeral stem loosening.

Allograft Prosthesis Composite Using Proximal Humeral Allograft

For many type 2 and type 3 bone defects, a proximal humeral allograft is an excellent option to address bone loss as well as lend structural support to the humeral stem (**Fig. 3**B). Benefits of a proximal humeral allograft include improved structural support of the component, restoration of humeral length and lateral offset, reconstitution of bone stock, and attachment sites for soft-tissue structures such as the posterior cuff, subscapularis, and deltoid.[4,20,21] Furthermore, in the setting of RTSA, the increased lateral offset provided by the allograft may be beneficial in improving the wrapping of the deltoid.[10,22]

After the previous humeral stem has been removed and bone loss has been more accurately assessed using trial implants, a proximal humeral allograft can be prepared for use. This is done by performing a cut at the anatomic neck of the allograft, just distal to the articular surface, which can be accomplished using a freehand technique or a cutting guide. The humeral canal is then reamed and broached, being sure to preserve enough cancellous bone for cement fixation. During this process, it is important to preserve the tendon stumps on the allograft for future repair to native tendons.[21]

An estimate regarding the length of allograft needed for reconstruction should be made preoperatively using radiographs with magnification markers, although final adjustments of stem height and size of allograft should be made intraoperatively based on total bone loss and soft-tissue tensioning. This can be accomplished either by overlying the humeral allograft on the native humerus with tension, or by using a long, loose-fitting broach in the native humerus to estimate size.[20] Once the length of allograft needed has been established, the distal humeral cut is made, which can include a step cut for added torsional stability.[4,21]

To achieve compression at the graft-host junction, a 3.5-mm locking compression plate may be used in compression mode across the junction, being sure to select a plate with adequate holes proximal and distal to the junction. Screws should be placed with a broach in place to ensure that the final cemented stem can pass into the canal; otherwise, cerclage wire at the site of the step cut may be used to achieve additional fixation.[20]

The broach can then be removed from the composite humerus and a cemented stem placed. The stem should be placed in the traditional 20° to 30° of retroversion, as this has been previously demonstrated to provide for the most optimal rotational ROM.[23] Any native tendons that have been preserved (posterior cuff, deltoid, pectoralis) should then be repaired to their respective allograft tendon stumps. If

the native subscapularis is still present, repair to the allograft tendon stump can be attempted to improve stability.[4,21]

Allograft Prosthesis Composite Using Femoral Strut Allograft

For longer diaphyseal bone defects (type 3B), one option for fixation is to use a femoral allograft. This is done by performing a "napkin ring" technique whereby a femoral allograft is cut to length to provide metaphyseal and diaphyseal structural support around the humeral stem (**Fig.** 3C). The advantages of this technique include the ease of application and the availability of the allograft.[12] Disadvantages include the lack of tendon stumps on the allograft for potential tendon repair. Furthermore, the clinical outcomes of this technique have not yet been reported.

Proximal Humeral or Total Humeral Replacement

Although more commonly used in the oncologic setting for wide resection of proximal humerus malignancies, a large proximal humeral endoprosthesis can be effectively used to span very large bone defects, such as PHAROS type 3B defects (**Fig.** 3D, E). The highly modular nature of these prostheses creates a relatively simple method of re-establishing humeral length; furthermore, proper version can normally be established through the modular components.[24] Native tendons can then be reattached to the prosthesis using suture fixation, although the healing of soft tissue to metal is questionable.

POSTOPERATIVE CARE

Postoperative rehabilitation protocols depend on the specific reconstruction technique used. Following implantation of an APC, most investigators recommend using a standard shoulder immobilizer for at least 6 weeks to allow for initial healing of the graft-host junction.[10,12,17] This can then be converted to a simple sling with gradual implementation of passive ROM exercises, such as pendulums. In general, any strengthening exercises should be avoided until 3 months postoperatively.

OUTCOMES

Proximal humeral bone loss has generally been associated with inferior outcomes because of poor stem fixation and difficulties in adequately restoring humeral length.[4,11] However, several studies have also demonstrated substantial clinical improvement with revision RTSA in the setting of proximal humeral bone loss, both with and without the use of structural allograft.[8,10,19,21,25] Furthermore, by achieving reliable humeral stem fixation, some studies have demonstrated no significant difference in outcomes between revision cases with and without proximal humeral bone loss.[8,25]

Several researchers have demonstrated good clinical results for revision RTSA with proximal humeral bone loss with a cemented humeral stem without an allograft. Budge and colleagues[19] performed revision RTSA with cemented stems in 15 patients with an average bone loss of 38.4 mm and found good clinical results at 2 years with no evidence of subsidence or loosening. The only prosthetic fracture observed was in a modular component, leading to a recommendation to only use monoblock humeral prostheses in this setting. Stephens and colleagues[8] reported significant improvement in clinical outcomes in patients with proximal humeral bone loss (average of 36.3 mm) converted from failed hemiarthroplasty to RTSA without the use of an allograft. The clinical results of these 16 patients with bone loss were equivalent to those patients without bone loss at the time of revision. However, humeral loosening was noted in 3 of these patients at final radiographic follow-up.[8]

Using a proximal humerus APC to address bone defects has been shown to be a reliable and effective means of achieving stability and improving clinical outcomes.[10,12,13,21,25,26] Chacon and colleagues[21] reported the 2-year clinical outcomes of 25 patients who underwent APC reconstruction for an average proximal humeral bone loss of 53.6 mm (34.5–150.3 mm) and demonstrated a significant improvement in ASES score (from 31.7 to 69.4) and Simple Shoulder Test score (from 1.4 to 4.5). Nineteen patients reported good to excellent results; only one patient had an unsatisfactory result. Patients' ROM improved in forward flexion (from 32.7° to 82.4°), abduction (from 40.4° to 81.4°), and internal rotation. Final radiographic follow-up demonstrated graft incorporation in the metaphysis in 84% of patients and in the diaphysis in 76% of patients.[21] Sanchez-Sotelo and colleagues[25] demonstrated similar clinical results in 26 patients treated with an APC at an average follow-up of 4 years.

There are limited data regarding proximal humeral replacements ("megaprostheses") or total humeral replacements. Guven and colleagues[24] performed a retrospective study of 10 patients who had undergone reverse shoulder tumor prosthesis placement for malignant proximal humerus tumors and reported low pain scores (mean visual analog score of 1.3) and satisfactory Disabilities of the Arm, Shoulder, and Hand scores (mean 26.2). The ROM at last follow-up was comparable with that of APC constructs, with an average forward flexion of 96° and active abduction of 88°.

SUMMARY

Although proximal humeral bone loss poses a significant obstacle to successful shoulder arthroplasty, viable reconstructive options are available to achieve stable humeral stem fixation and restore humeral length. Using a systematic evaluation of bone loss both preoperatively and intraoperatively for surgical decision making, satisfactory patient outcomes can be expected with either cemented stem fixation or an APC construct. In cases of catastrophic bone loss, proximal and total humeral prostheses are a reasonable option.

REFERENCES

1. Kim SH, Wise BL, Zhang Y, et al. Increasing incidence of shoulder arthroplasty in the United States. J Bone Joint Surg Am 2011;93(24):2249–54.
2. Sershon RA, Van Thiel GS, Lin EC, et al. Clinical outcomes of reverse total shoulder arthroplasty in patients aged younger than 60 years. J Shoulder Elbow Surg 2014;23(3):395–400.
3. Zumstein MA, Pinedo M, Old J, et al. Problems, complications, reoperations, and revisions in reverse total shoulder arthroplasty: a systematic review. J Shoulder Elbow Surg 2011;20(1):146–57.
4. Boileau P. Complications and revision of reverse total shoulder arthroplasty. Orthop Traumatol Surg Res 2016;102(1 Suppl):S33–43.
5. Wall B, Nove-Josserand L, O'Connor DP, et al. Reverse total shoulder arthroplasty: a review of results according to etiology. J Bone Joint Surg Am 2007;89(7):1476–85.
6. Black EM, Roberts SM, Siegel E, et al. Reverse shoulder arthroplasty as salvage for failed prior arthroplasty in patients 65 years of age or younger. J Shoulder Elbow Surg 2014;23(7):1036–42.
7. Jones RB, Wright TW, Zuckerman JD. Reverse total shoulder arthroplasty with structural bone grafting of large glenoid defects. J Shoulder Elbow Surg 2016;25(9):1425–32.
8. Stephens SP, Paisley KC, Giveans MR, et al. The effect of proximal humeral bone loss on revision reverse total shoulder arthroplasty. J Shoulder Elbow Surg 2015;24(10):1519–26.
9. Holcomb JO, Cuff D, Petersen SA, et al. Revision reverse shoulder arthroplasty for glenoid baseplate

failure after primary reverse shoulder arthroplasty. J Shoulder Elbow Surg 2009;18(5):717–23.

10. Levy J, Frankle M, Mighell M, et al. The use of the reverse shoulder prosthesis for the treatment of failed hemiarthroplasty for proximal humeral fracture. J Bone Joint Surg Am 2007;89(2):292–300.

11. Cuff D, Levy JC, Gutierrez S, et al. Torsional stability of modular and non-modular reverse shoulder humeral components in a proximal humeral bone loss model. J Shoulder Elbow Surg 2011;20(4): 646–51.

12. Chalmers PN, Boileau P, Romeo AA, et al. Revision reverse shoulder arthroplasty. J Am Acad Orthop Surg 2019;27(12):426–36.

13. McLendon PB, Cox JL, Frankle MA. Humeral bone loss in revision shoulder arthroplasty. Am J Orthop (Belle Mead NJ) 2018;47(2). https://doi.org/10.12788/ajo.2018.0012.

14. Chalmers PN, Romeo AA, Nicholson GP, et al. Humeral bone loss in revision total shoulder arthroplasty: the proximal humeral arthroplasty revision osseous insufficiency (PHAROS) classification system. Clin Orthop Relat Res 2019;477(2):432–41.

15. Cil A, Veillette CJ, Sanchez-Sotelo J, et al. Survivorship of the humeral component in shoulder arthroplasty. J Shoulder Elbow Surg 2010;19(1):143–50.

16. Raiss P, Edwards TB, Deutsch A, et al. Radiographic changes around humeral components in shoulder arthroplasty. J Bone Joint Surg Am 2014;96(7):e54.

17. Petkovic D, Kovacevic D, Levine WN, et al. Management of the failed arthroplasty for proximal humerus fracture. J Am Acad Orthop Surg 2019;27(2): 39–49.

18. Van Thiel GS, Halloran JP, Twigg S, et al. The vertical humeral osteotomy for stem removal in revision shoulder arthroplasty: results and technique. J Shoulder Elbow Surg 2011;20(8):1248–54.

19. Budge MD, Moravek JE, Zimel MN, et al. Reverse total shoulder arthroplasty for the management of failed shoulder arthroplasty with proximal humeral bone loss: is allograft augmentation necessary? J Shoulder Elbow Surg 2013;22(6): 739–44.

20. Sanchez-Sotelo J, Wagner ER, Houdek MT. Allograft-prosthetic composite reconstruction for massive proximal humeral bone loss in reverse shoulder arthroplasty. JBJS Essent Surg Tech 2018;8(1):e3.

21. Chacon A, Virani N, Shannon R, et al. Revision arthroplasty with use of a reverse shoulder prosthesis-allograft composite. J Bone Joint Surg Am 2009;91(1):119–27.

22. Gagey O, Hue E. Mechanics of the deltoid muscle. A new approach. Clin Orthop Relat Res 2000;(375): 250–7.

23. Rhee YG, Cho NS, Moon SC. Effects of humeral component retroversion on functional outcomes in reverse total shoulder arthroplasty for cuff tear arthropathy. J Shoulder Elbow Surg 2015;24(10): 1574–81.

24. Guven MF, Aslan L, Botanlioglu H, et al. Functional outcome of reverse shoulder tumor prosthesis in the treatment of proximal humerus tumors. J Shoulder Elbow Surg 2016;25(1):e1–6.

25. Sanchez-Sotelo J, Wagner ER, Sim FH, et al. Allograft-prosthetic composite reconstruction for massive proximal humeral bone loss in reverse shoulder arthroplasty. J Bone Joint Surg Am 2017; 99(24):2069–76.

26. McLendon PB, Cox JL, Frankle MA. Large diaphyseal-incorporating allograft prosthetic composites: when, how, and why : treatment of advanced proximal humeral bone loss. Orthopade 2017;46(12):1022–7.

Osteochondral Reconstruction of the Capitellum

Brent J. Morris, MD[a],*, Casey J. Kiser, MD[a],
Hussein A. Elkousy, MD[a], J. Michael Bennett, MD[b],
Thomas L. Mehlhoff, MD[a]

KEYWORDS

- Osteochondritis dissecans • Capitellum • Osteochondral reconstruction • OATS

KEY POINTS

- Osteochondritis dissecans of the capitellum is a localized inflammatory condition in adolescent patients who participate in repetitive overhead sports and upper extremity weightbearing activities.
- Lesions can be described as stable or unstable depending on the stability of the articular surface, with stable lesions being susceptible to nonoperative treatment and unstable lesions necessitating surgical intervention.
- Various surgical interventions have been described including drilling of the lesion, fragment excision with drilling, fragment fixation, reconstruction with autograft plug, autologous chondrocyte implantation, and closing wedge osteotomy.
- The posterior anconeus muscle splitting approach to elbow with reconstruction of the lesion using an autograft plug from the ipsilateral knee is our preferred treatment for an unstable lesion failing nonoperative treatment.

INTRODUCTION

Osteochondritis dissecans (OCD) of the capitellum, first described by König in 1888,[1] is an idiopathic, localized inflammatory pathologic condition affecting the subchondral bone and overlying cartilage in the capitellum. The exact cause is unknown; however, this injury is most commonly attributed to repetitive microtrauma from valgus compression-type injuries of the immature capitellar articular cartilage causing vascular insufficiency. Ultimately, localized necrosis and subchondral bone changes can occur, with cartilage fragmentation after loss of mechanical support.[2,3] Loss of articular cartilage from the donor site and mechanical wear from the loose body can lead to early arthritic changes. Genetic predisposition to this injury may be possible; however, this is as yet unconfirmed.

CAUSE

- Largely unknown, multiple theories
- Repetitive mechanical trauma
- Disruption of blood supply to small areas of the bone
- Disruption of enchondral ossification

OCD of the capitellum is a fairly uncommon condition with an incidence of 2.2 per 100,000 in adolescent patients.[4] It is most often seen in patients aged 12 to 16 years who participate

[a] Fondren Orthopaedic Group, TERFSES Shoulder and Elbow Fellowship, Texas Orthopedic Hospital, 7401 South Main Street, Houston, TX 77030, USA; [b] Fondren Orthopaedic Group, 7401 South Main Street, Houston, TX 77030, USA
* Corresponding author.
E-mail address: brent.joseph.morris@gmail.com

Orthop Clin N Am 51 (2020) 97–108
https://doi.org/10.1016/j.ocl.2019.08.004
0030-5898/20/© 2019 Elsevier Inc. All rights reserved.

in repetitive overhead sports and upper extremity weightbearing activities, with baseball and football players, as well as gymnasts, being the most commonly affected patients.[4] Often, this is seen in the dominant extremity and has a higher prevalence in boys with a boy:girl ratio of 6.4:1.[4]

Most often these patients present with insidious, activity-related elbow pain on the lateral aspect of the elbow in the dominant arm.[5] Common complaints include mechanical symptoms and or loss of full extension.[5] The patient may complain of catching or locking symptoms in advanced disease with loose bodies. On physical examination, the patient typically has lateral elbow tenderness to palpation, a small effusion, and mild loss of extension, as well crepitus or catching with range of motion in advanced disease.

SYMPTOMS

- Elbow pain with activity, relieved with rest
- Loss of motion, especially loss of full extension
- Swelling
- Mechanical symptoms such as grinding, catching, locking, and clicking

PHYSICAL EXAMINATION FINDINGS

- Tenderness laterally
- Loss of extension
- Swelling

IMAGING

Patients who present with clinical examination findings and subjective history consistent with that of an OCD lesion should initially have an anteroposterior (AP) and lateral radiograph of the elbow to evaluate for any irregular ossification or bony defects (Fig. 1). In addition, a 45° AP flexion view[6] can be helpful. Contralateral elbow radiographs can be valuable for comparative imaging. In more advanced disease, a crater of rarefaction in the capitellum may be present and usually has a sclerotic rim of subchondral bone adjacent to the articular surface.[7] Advanced imaging is often indicated to better identify and classify the lesion. We prefer both a computerized tomography (CT) and an MRI scan in these cases. A CT scan is essential in defining the bony anatomy underlying the cartilage defect and to look for loose bodies, whereas an MRI is ideal to assess the extent of the osteochondritis and determine if a lesion is unstable (Fig. 2). We also perform an AP or

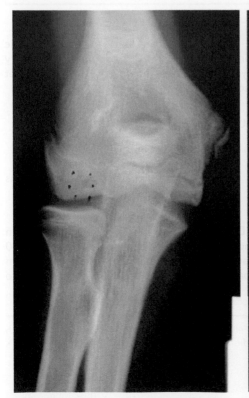
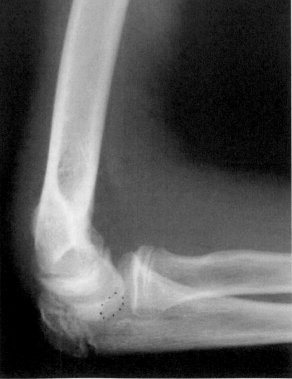

Fig. 1. AP and lateral radiographs of the elbow with the osteochrondral defect of the capitellum outlined.

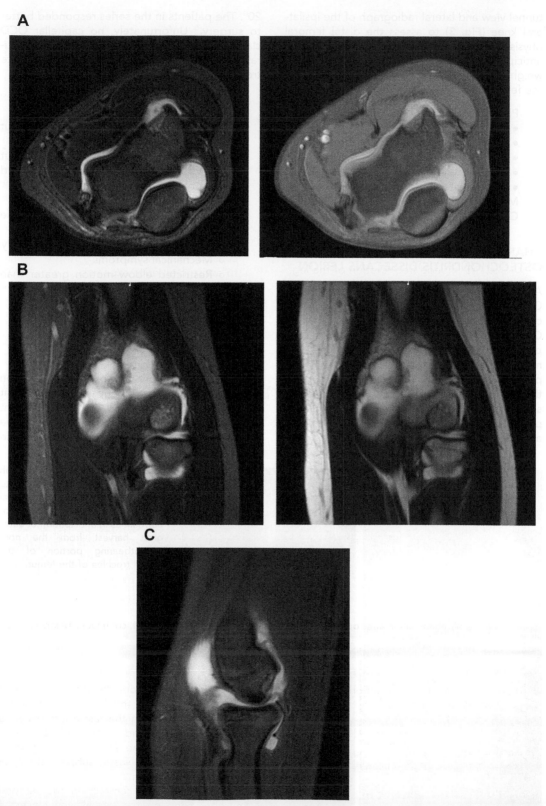

Fig. 2. (A) T1 and T2 MRI axial images showing a large unstable osteochondral defect of the capitellum. (B) T1 and T2 MRI coronal images showing a large unstable osteochondral defect of the capitellum. (C) T2 MRI axial image showing a large unstable osteochondral defect of the capitellum.

tunnel view and lateral radiograph of the ipsilateral knee (**Fig. 3**) to assess the distal femoral
physis and rule out any bony abnormalities in
anticipation of autograft harvest from the non-
weightbearing portion of the lateral trochlea of
the femur.

    Plain radiographs
    - AP
    - Lateral
    - 45° AP flexion view[6]
    - Contralateral elbow views for comparison
    - AP and lateral of the ipsilateral knee
    MRI
    CT

CHARACTERIZING THE OSTEOCHONDRITIS DISSECANS LESION

Although there are multiple classifications of
OCD lesions of the elbow, the Takahara classification is most commonly used.[6] Stable capitellar
OCD lesions were defined in patients with open
physes, low-grade radiographic changes, and
maintained range of motion of the elbow. These
patients responded to nonoperative measures in
the reported series.[6] Unstable capitellar OCD lesions were defined in patients with closed
physes, higher-grade radiographic changes,
and restriction of elbow motion greater than

20°. The patients in the series responded better
to surgery.[6] Unfortunately, no capitellar OCD
classification system has been shown to accurately predict healing or direct appropriate
treatment.

- Stable lesion—articular cartilage intact
  ○ Open growth plates
  ○ Normal elbow motion without
    mechanical elbow symptoms
  ○ Radiographic lucency without
    fragmentation or loose body visualized
    on plain films
  ○ MRI reveals intact articular cartilage
- Unstable lesion "in situ"—unstable
  cartilage flap
- Unstable lesion "displaced"—loose body
  ○ Mechanical symptoms
  ○ Restricted elbow motion greater than
    20°
  ○ Closing or closed physis
  ○ Failed nonoperative management

TREATMENT

The treatment approach for this uncommon
problem ranges from nonoperative treatment
in stable lesions to various surgical treatment
options. Many surgical treatment options have
been described including microfracture, loose

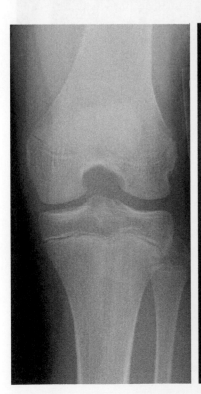 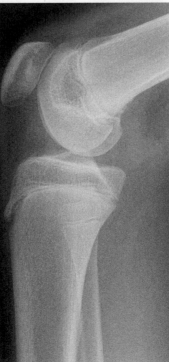

Fig. 3. AP and lateral radiograph
of the knee. It is necessary to
assess the distal femoral
physis and rule out any bony abnormalities in anticipation of autograft harvest from the non-
weightbearing portion of the
lateral trochlea of the femur.

body removal, abrasion chondroplasty, lesion fixation, isolated osteochondral allograft transplantation surgery (OATS), autologous chondrocyte implantation, lateral condyle closing wedge osteotomy and OATS for larger, unstable lesions. Our preferred surgical treatment option for unstable OCD lesions of the capitellum is a novel surgical technique with osteochondral autologous transplantation surgery using an autograft from the ipsilateral knee.

Stable OCD lesion
- Rest
- Cessation of the repetitive stress across the elbow
- Stretching and strengthening exercises
- Return to activities when pain free and radiographs confirm a healed lesion

Unstable OCD lesion
- Surgical intervention
  ○ Drilling of the lesion
  ○ Fragment removal with or without curettage or drilling of the residual defect
  ○ Fragment fixation by a variety of methods
  ○ Reconstruction with osteochondral autograft (knee)—our preferred technique
  ○ Autologous chondrocyte implantation
  ○ Closing wedge osteotomy of the lateral condyle

INDICATIONS/CONTRAINDICATIONS

The primary indication for surgical intervention for an OCD of the capitellum reconstruction with an OATS procedure includes larger unstable lesions of the capitellum (usually 8–12 mm). Contraindications for surgical treatment of OCD lesions of the capitellum include stable lesions, traumatic cartilage shear injuries, and Panner disease. Panner disease is osteochondrosis of the capitellum that occurs primarily in young boys under 10 years and can often be confused with OCD of the capitellum. Panner disease is a self-limiting condition that is treated nonoperatively. Atypically large size may be a relative contraindication for our particular autograft procedure because the largest bone harvester is 10 mm. Atypically large OCD lesions can be potentially treated with a combination of 2 autograft plugs; however, this is not our preferred treatment option given concern for possible inconsistent healing when using 2 plugs. Our preferred treatment method for larger defects (>10 mm in

diameter) is to apply the autograft to the area of most concern within the lesion.

Indications
Unstable Lesions
Lesions not responding to conservative measures

Contraindications
Stable lesions
Panner disease (osteochondrosis of the capitellum)
Traumatic cartilage shear injuries
Size too large (>10 mm) is a relative contraindication for autograft, given that 10 mm is the largest bone harvester/autograft plug size, but placement of the graft in the area of most concern is a viable treatment option.

Surgical technique/procedure
Preoperative planning. Preoperative planning must include performance of all relevant imaging, including radiographs (elbow and ipsilateral knee), CT, and MRI as noted above once the patient has been deemed a surgical candidate for capitellar OATS. Coordination is key to the intraoperative plan between the elbow specialist and the knee specialist for knee autograft harvesting.

Preparation and patient positioning. The patient is placed in the supine position with an arm table (**Fig. 4**). The ipsilateral leg is left exposed. The patient is anesthetized with general anesthesia. No peripheral nerve blocks are performed. A nonsterile tourniquet is placed on both the upper and lower extremity. The entire arm and leg are prepped and draped (**Fig. 5**). The procedure can be performed

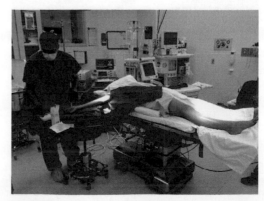

Fig. 4. The patient is placed in the supine position with an arm table and the ipsilateral leg left exposed.

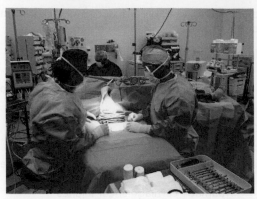

Fig. 5. The entire arm and leg are prepped and draped. Nonsterile tourniquets are placed on both the upper and lower extremities.

simultaneously with a second surgeon for autograft harvest from the knee once proper sizing of the capitellar OCD lesion has been determined. Alternatively, in the absence of a knee surgeon for autograft harvest from the knee, the surgeon can start with exposure of elbow and transition to the knee for harvest once proper sizing of the lesion has been determined.

Surgical approach elbow and host site preparation. The upper extremity tourniquet is insufflated at 200 mm Hg. Our technique is a posterior anconeus muscle-splitting approach, originally described by Iwasaki and colleagues.[8] A 4.5-cm oblique incision is used at the posterior aspect of the flexed operative elbow from the ulnar shaft to the lateral epicondyle using the ulnar shaft, lateral epicondyle, and ulnar tip as the 3 key bony landmarks (**Fig. 6**). The skin is incised while the elbow is in full flexion (**Fig. 7**).

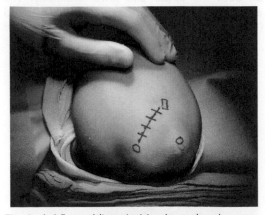

Fig. 6. A 4.5-cm oblique incision is used at the posterior aspect of the flexed operative elbow from the ulnar shaft to the lateral epicondyle, using the ulnar shaft, lateral epicondyle, and ulnar tip as the 3 key bony landmarks.

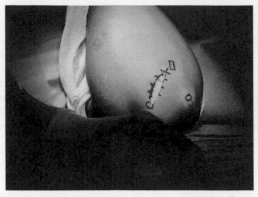

Fig. 7. Skin incision is made with the elbow in full flexion.

Subcutaneous tissue is divided to expose the fascia of the anconeus muscle. The fascia is incised longitudinally. The anconeus is spread to expose the posterior capsule (**Fig. 8**), which is incised longitudinally to enter the joint (**Fig. 9**). The joint is examined for any synovitis, which is sharply resected if present. At this point the articular cartilage over the capitellum is visualized and closely scrutinized. The unstable flap of articular cartilage is sharply resected to expose the lesion (**Fig. 10**). The margins of the lesion are sharply debrided to ensure only normal cartilage remains. The lesion is then sized using sizing guides to determine the best match for the defect (**Fig. 11**). Core decompression of the lesion is begun at this point first by inserting the matching harvester sizing cylinder (**Fig. 12**). The proper-sized cannulated sizing cylinder is placed into the defect and the guide pin is inserted through the sizing cylinder. The sizing

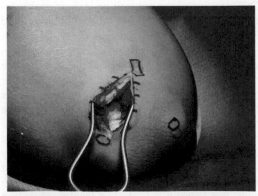

Fig. 8. The approach starts with dividing the subcutaneous tissue to expose the fascia of the anconeus muscle. The fascia is incised longitudinally. The anconeus is spread to expose the posterior capsule.

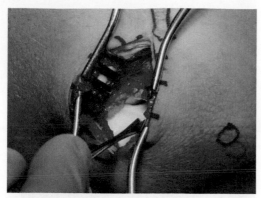

Fig. 9. The posterior capsule is incised longitudinally to enter the joint. A freer is marking the unstable cartilage lesion.

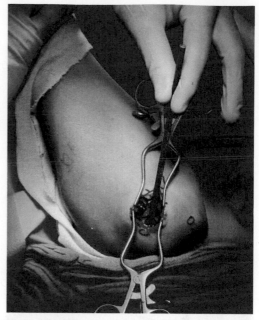

Fig. 11. The capitellar OCD lesion is sized using sizing guides to determine the best match for the defect.

cylinder ensures that the guide pin is centered within the defect and perpendicular to the defect (**Fig. 13**). This is confirmed with visual inspection. Attention is then turned to autograft harvest from the knee.

Elbow Approach and Host Site Preparation

1. A 4.5-cm oblique incision with the elbow in full flexion
2. Expose the anconeus fascia and incise longitudinally
3. Elbow joint capsule is exposed and incised longitudinally to enter the joint
4. Sharply debride any synovitis, remove loose bodies, and excise the unstable flap
5. Determine the size of the defect with the sizing guide
6. Place a guide pin for core decompression using the proper-sized cannulated sizing cylinder and visually confirm the guide pin is centered with the lesion

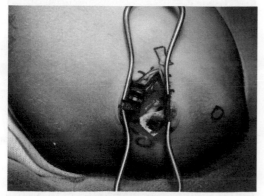

Fig. 10. The unstable flap of articular cartilage is sharply resected to expose the capitellar OCD lesion. The margins of the OCD lesion are sharply debrided to ensure that only normal cartilage remains.

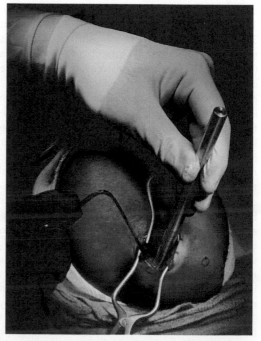

Fig. 12. Core decompression of the lesion is completed at this point first by inserting the matching harvester sizing cylinder. The proper-sized cannulated sizing cylinder is placed into the defect and the guide pin is inserted through the sizing cylinder.

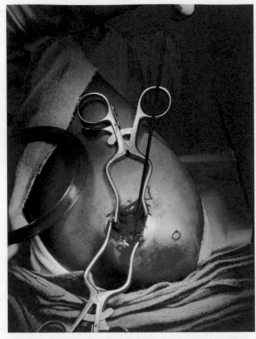

Fig. 13. The sizing cylinder ensures that the guide pin is centered within the defect and perpendicular to the defect.

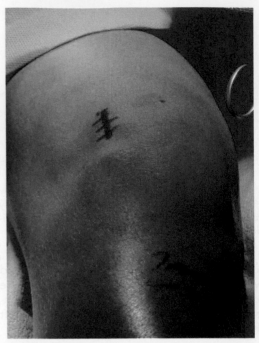

Fig. 14. The graft harvest is performed through a 5-cm longitudinal incision made on the lateral aspect of the patella.

Surgical approach ipsilateral knee and autograft harvesting. Attention is then turned to autograft harvest from the ipsilateral knee. The lower extremity tourniquet is insufflated at 300 mm Hg and a 5-cm longitudinal incision is made on the lateral aspect of the patella (**Fig. 14**). Dissection is performed down to the superficial retinaculum, which is then split perpendicular to its fibers. The deep retinaculum is then identified and split. The capsule is identified and sharply split vertically to expose the lateral trochlea. At this point the OATS harvester is placed proximal to the sulcus terminalis in the non-weightbearing articular surface of the lateral trochlea of the knee and the graft is subsequently harvested. The diameter of the plug is based on the size of the capitellar lesion; however, the depth depends on the proximity of the graft harvest site to the physis. The typical harvest depth is around 10–12 mm; however, this may be modified if the location of the harvest is near the physis. The harvest site is then remeasured and an allograft plug, oversized by 1 mm in diameter, is used to fill the defect (**Fig. 15**) and impacted into place ensuring the graft is flush with the surrounding articular surface.

1. Approach to the non-weightbearing portion of the lateral trochlea of the ipsilateral knee

2. Graft harvester is used to extract the autograft of the proper size and to a depth that safely avoids the physis
3. A size-matched allograft plug is placed to backfill the knee harvest site

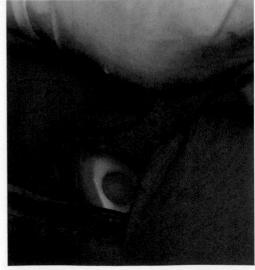

Fig. 15. An allograft plug is used to backfill the donor site defect ensuring that the graft is placed flush with the surrounding articular surface.

Core decompression and autograft insertion. Attention is turned back to the capitellum. The cannulated reamer corresponding to the diameter of the defect is then passed over the previously placed guide pin, removing dead bone with a core decompression to a depth typically around 10–12 mm; however, this is altered based on the autograft depth harvested from the knee (**Fig. 16**). The sizing cylinder is placed into the reamed defect to confirm the depth of the defect. The core decompression site is closely examined to ensure that healthy cancellous bone remains and that there is healthy surrounding articular cartilage.

The autograft plug is then brought to the elbow and fashioned with a rongeur to address any high or low areas and to match the proper depth. The autograft plug is oriented with the high side to the lateral direction to match the native anatomy. The harvester is then positioned at the site of the core decompression site and the graft is advanced into the previously reamed channel (**Fig. 17**). The graft is initially left 2–3 mm proud (**Fig. 18**) after being deployed from the harvester, and then final tapping of the graft is performed with the sizers to ensure

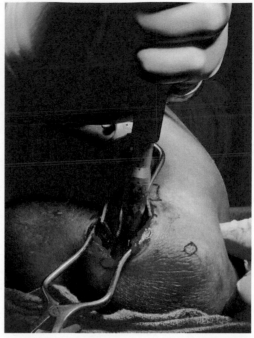

Fig. 17. The autograft plug is oriented with the high side to the lateral direction to match the native anatomy. The harvester is then positioned at the site of the core decompression site and the graft is advanced into the previously reamed channel.

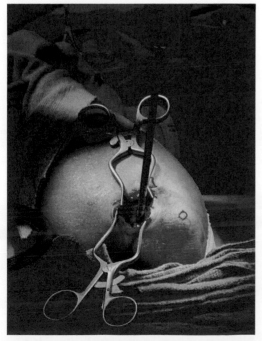

Fig. 16. The cannulated reamer corresponding to the size of the defect is passed over the guide pin, removing dead bone with a core decompression to a depth typically around 10–12 mm depending on the size of the autograft plug harvested from the knee.

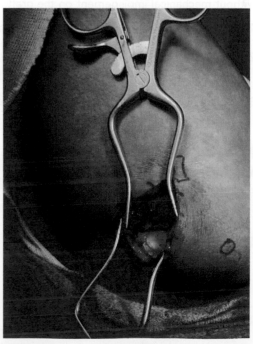

Fig. 18. The graft is initially left 2–3 mm proud after being deployed from the harvester.

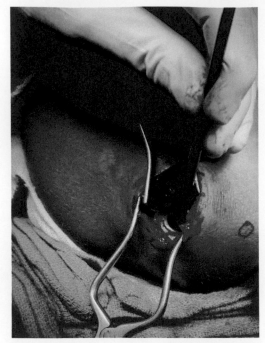

Fig. 19. Final tapping of the graft is performed with the sizers to ensure a perfect match with the articular cartilage of the capitellum.

a perfect match with the articular cartilage of the capitellum (**Figs. 19** and **20**). Range of motion is assessed after final graft seating to ensure full flexion, extension, pronation, and supination without mechanical impingement on the graft.

1. Autograft plug is fashioned with rongeur and depth is noted
2. Ream over the guide pin with the size-matched cannulated reamer to the proper depth and remove the guide pin
3. Graft is deployed into the core decompression site by advancing the graft

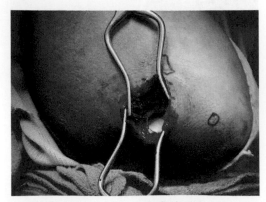

Fig. 20. Final autograft implant flush with surrounding articular surface.

with the harvester and initially leave 2–3 mm proud
4. Final insertion of the graft using sizer as an impactor
5. Ensure the graft is perfectly flush with the articular surface
6. Confirm elbow range of motion and no mechanical impingement on the graft

Surgical wound closure
Both surgical wounds are thoroughly irrigated. The elbow capsule is closed with interrupted nonabsorbable 3-0 suture with the knots buried. The anconeus muscle is allowed to fall back into position and the overlying fascia is closed with interrupted nonabsorbable 3-0 sutures with the knots buried (**Fig. 21**). The overlying skin is closed with a deep absorbable 4-0 suture and a subcutaneous absorbable 5-0 subcuticular running suture, followed by interrupted 6-0 nylon sutures for the skin. The wound is dressed and the patient is placed in a well-padded posterior slab splint in 90° of flexion and neutral rotation.

The knee closure begins with the deep portion of the retinaculum being only partially closed to prevent lateral patellar compression syndrome. The superficial retinaculum is also left open. The deep skin layer is closed with an

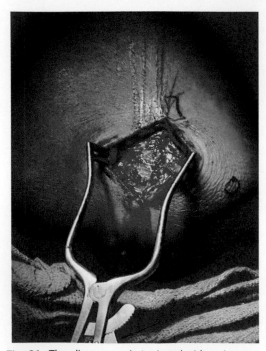

Fig. 21. The elbow capsule is closed with an interrupted nonabsorbable 3-0 suture with the knots buried. The anconeus muscle is allowed to fall back into position and the overlying fascia is closed with interrupted nonabsorbable 3-0 sutures with the knots buried.

absorbable suture with the superficial skin closed with a running subcuticular absorbable suture. A soft sterile dressing is applied. No bracing or splint is used for the knee.

COMPLICATIONS

- Infection
- Graft failure
- Nerve symptoms
- Contracture
- Recurrent loose bodies
- Donor site pain
- Recurrent mechanical pain

Complications following this procedure are rare, but those to consider include infection, graft failure, nerve symptoms, contracture, recurrent loose bodies, donor site pain, and recurrence of mechanical symptoms. Fortunately, complications in our patient series have been rare. One patient did experience painless crepitus at the radiocapitellar joint despite excellent radiographic appearance, otherwise no other complications have been reported to date in our small series.

Elbow Postoperative Care

At 1 week postoperatively the elbow splint is removed and a removable splint is placed at 90°, and the patient is allowed to begin a gentle range of motion protocol at home. At 2 weeks postoperatively, the nylon sutures are removed and the patient is placed in a range of motion elbow brace with continued focus on range of motion for 6 weeks and allowing full elbow range of motion in the brace. At 8 weeks postoperatively, elbow radiographs are obtained to ensure healing of the graft, and elbow strengthening can start 12 weeks postoperatively. The patient is progressed in their activity to tolerance, but specifically restricted from doing push-ups and resisted elbow extension. Return to sport is typically allowed at the 6-month postoperative time frame.

Knee Postoperative Care

Regarding the knee, the postoperative protocol includes initially allowing the patient to be weightbearing as tolerated. The authors encourage the patient to do home exercises including quadriceps sets and heel slides. After the first postoperative knee appointment at the 2-week mark, the patient is allowed to begin using a stationary bike and progress to low-impact activities for 6 to 8 weeks postoperatively. We allow the patient to gradually transition to running, jumping, and high-impact activities at around the 3-month postoperative mark.

Outcomes

Preliminary data from our center following OATS autograft from the ipsilateral knee for an unstable OCD lesion of the capitellum include 16 adolescent athletes (14 boys and 2 girls) with an average age of 14.2 years (12–16 years) and 1-year minimum follow-up. Autograft plug sizes were 6,[2] 8,[7] and 10 mm.[7] Thirteen patients had excellent results using a modified Timmerman and Andrews scoring system,[9] 2 patients had a good result, and 1 patient had a fair result (painless radiocapitellar crepitus as noted above). Range of motion improved in all patients with symmetric range of motion noted in all patients at final follow-up. There were no intraoperative elbow or knee complications in our series. Two patients did have further elbow surgery unrelated to their OATS procedure. One patient had an elbow arthroscopy 4 years after OATS for recurrent elbow joint synovitis, and one patient had an ulnar collateral ligament reconstruction 4 years after OATS. There were no other postoperative elbow complications. There were *no* reported complications secondary to the ipsilateral knee harvest site. There were no revision surgeries secondary to graft malpositioning, dislocation, or recurrent OCD lesions.

SUMMARY

OCD lesions of the capitellum are uncommon, but can occur in adolescents, especially athletes in overhead sports. Our preferred surgical technique for the treatment of unstable OCD lesions of the capitellum is osteochondral autologous transplantation surgery using autograft from the ipsilateral knee. The authors prefer a supine position and a posterior anconeus muscle splitting approach with the elbow in flexion to address the capitellar OCD lesion. We have been pleased with our series of patients using this approach with minimal complications and excellent early outcomes.

REFERENCES

1. Churchill R, Munoz K, Ahmad C. Osteochondritis dissecans of the elbow. Curr Rev Musculoskelet Med 2016;9(2):232–9.
2. Douglas G, Rang M. The role of trauma in the pathogenesis of the osteochondrosis. Clin Orthop Relat Res 1981;158:28–32.
3. Takahara M, Ogino T, Takagi M, et al. Natural progression of the osteochondritis dissecans of the humeral capitellum: initial observations. Radiology 2000;216:207–12.

4. Kessler J, Jacobs J, Cannamela P, et al. Demographics and epidemiology of osteochondritis dissecans of the elbow among children and adolescents. Orthop J Sports Med 2018;6(12). 2325967118815846.

5. McManama G, Michel L, Berry MV, et al. The surgical treatment of osteochondritis of the capitellum. Am J Sports Med 1985;13(1):11–21.

6. Takahara M, Mura N, Sasaki J, et al. Classification, treatment, and outcome of osteochondritis dissecans of the humeral capitellum. J Bone Joint Surg Am 2007;89(6):1205–14.

7. Shaughnessy WJ. Osteochondritis dissecans. In: Morrey BF, Sanchez-Sotelo J, Morrey ME, editors. Morrey's the elbow and its disorders. 5th edition. Philadelphia: Elsevier; 2018. p. 341–8.

8. Iwasaki N, Kato H, Ishikawa J, et al. Autologous osteochondral mosaicplasty for osteochondritis dissecans of the elbow in teenage athletes. J Bone Joint Surg Am 2009;91(10):2359–66.

9. Timmerman LA, Andrews JR. Arthroscopic treatment of posttraumatic elbow pain and stiffness. Am J Sports Med 1994;22:230–5.

Foot and Ankle

Outcomes of Reconstruction of the Flexible Adult-acquired Flatfoot Deformity

Matthew S. Conti, MD[a], Jonathan H. Garfinkel, MD[b],
Scott J. Ellis, MD[c],*

KEYWORDS

• Adult-acquired flatfoot deformity • Patient-reported outcomes • Reconstruction

KEY POINTS

- Reconstruction of the flexible adult-acquired flatfoot deformity typically includes a combination of a flexor digitorum longus transfer, medializing calcaneal osteotomy (MCO), heel cord lengthening/gastrocnemius recession, lateral column lengthening (LCL), Cotton osteotomy or first tarsometatarsal fusion, and spring ligament reconstruction.
- When performing an MCO, the optimal heel position as measured by the hindfoot moment arm is between 0 mm and 5 mm of varus, or a clinically straight heel.
- LCL is often used to correct the midfoot abduction deformity; however, overcorrection of the talonavicular joint into a position of adduction may to lead to inferior postoperative patient-reported outcomes.
- Excessive plantarflexion of the medial cuneiform after a Cotton osteotomy has been correlated with worse postoperative clinical outcomes and should be avoided. The Cotton osteotomy should not be used to compensate for excessive residual supination occurring along the medial arch at locations other than the medial cuneiform.
- Reconstruction of flexible flatfeet in obese and older patients is an acceptable alternative to arthrodesis.

INTRODUCTION

Adult-acquired flatfoot deformity (AAFD) encompasses numerous individual deformities of the foot, including hindfoot valgus, forefoot abduction, sag at the talonavicular joint, and forefoot varus or supination.[1] Although the prevalence of symptomatic AAFD is not known, 1 study estimated that 3.3% of women over the age of 40 years old are affected.[2] AAFD can be debilitating and, among foot and ankle disorders, is second only to ankle arthritis in severity of preoperative pain and limitation in physical function as assessed by patient-reported Patient-Reported Outcomes Measurement Information System (PROMIS) outcome scores.[3]

As the ligaments, tendons, and bony structures that support the talus fail, there is a progressive deformity of the foot and ankle leading to AAFD.[1,4] The classification system originally developed for posterior tibial tendon deficiency (PTTD) has been applied to AAFD, and each stage from I to IV requires a different approach to management.[1,5] Stage II PTTD

Disclosure Statement: The authors have nothing to disclose.
[a] Hospital for Special Surgery, 535 East 70th Street, New York, NY 10021, USA; [b] Cedars-Sinai Medical Center, 444 S. San Vicente Boulevard, Suite 603, Los Angeles, CA 90048, USA; [c] Department of Orthopaedic Foot and Ankle Surgery, Hospital for Special Surgery, 535 East 70th Street, New York, NY 10021, USA
* Corresponding author.
E-mail address: elliss@hss.edu

Orthop Clin N Am 51 (2020) 109–120
https://doi.org/10.1016/j.ocl.2019.08.005

consists of patients with flexible hindfoot valgus and forefoot abduction deformities and is the most controversial in terms of surgical treatment.[6] These patients often benefit from reconstruction of their deformities, unlike patients in stage I, who typically are managed nonoperatively, and those in stage III, who have rigid deformities that are better treated with arthrodesis.[1,5] As patients move from stage I to stage IV, the deformities typically become more difficult to treat, and the outcomes of surgical management decline.[5] Therefore, tailoring a flatfoot reconstruction for stage II PTTD, or flexible AAFD, to an individual patient's deformity has been the subject of significant research over the past 2 decades. This article summarizes the literature on outcomes of reconstruction of the flexible AAFD in order to help the orthopedic surgeon understand advances in surgical techniques.

CLINICAL OUTCOMES IN FLEXIBLE ADULT-ACQUIRED FLATFOOT DEFORMITY
Evaluation of Adult-acquired Flatfoot Deformity
Clinical examination of the patient with AAFD begins with assessing the severity of the sag at the talonavicular joint, hindfoot valgus, and medial arch supination deformities. More severe AAFD can present with talar tilt at the ankle due insufficiency of the deltoid ligament. On physical examination, inability to perform a single-heel raise suggests deficiency of the posterior tibial tendon. The test is performed by having the patient balance on 1 foot and then lift the ipsilateral heel off the ground. The single-heel raise test is positive when the patient cannot raise the heel off the ground or when normal heel inversion is absent.[1] Calluses along the medial arch of the foot suggest collapse of the medial longitudinal arch and occur because these patients do not reconstitute their arch during heel-toe progression. The talar head may be palpated at the talonavicular joint, and the examiner can evaluate whether the sag at the talonavicular joint is flexible. The severity of forefoot abduction should be judged clinically, and the too many toes sign, where the clinician stands behind the patient and judges whether more toes than typical are seen lateral to the heel, may be exacerbated by the abduction and/or valgus hindfoot deformity. It is important for the examiner to determine if forefoot abduction is flexible or rigid because this guides treatment. Forefoot varus can be assessed by applying pressure to the fourth and fifth metatarsals as the ankle is dorsiflexed

with the hindfoot in neutral and evaluating the elevation of the first metatarsal with respect to the fifth metatarsal.[7] In patients who have an unstable first ray, dorsiflexing and plantarflexing the first ray with the other metatarsals stabilized may reveal excessive motion and painful crepitus at the first tarsometatarsal (TMT) joint.[7] Patients with AAFD frequently have gastrocnemius or Achilles tendon tightness, and this can be addressed if the patient undergoes surgery. With hindfoot valgus corrected, the surgeon should perform the Silfverskiold test to determine if the patient's ankle dorsiflexion improves with knee flexion, suggesting isolated gastrocnemius tightness, which can be managed with gastrocnemius lengthening alone.[1] If knee flexion does not improve ankle dorsiflexion, then the patient has Achilles tendon tightness and should be treated with a tendo-Achilles lengthening. To properly perform the Silfverskiold test in patients with flexible AAFD, correction of hindfoot valgus is necessary, otherwise dorsiflexion motion occurs in an oblique plane through the transverse tarsal and subtalar joints.[8] Patients with stage II PTTD have a flexible deformity, which includes adequate motion at the subtalar joint. For these patients, physical examination demonstrates proper inversion of the heels during a successful double heel rise.

Outcomes of flexible AAFD have often been correlated to improvements in radiographic parameters. Although documenting clinical changes in hindfoot position is useful, it tends to underestimate the bony valgus deformity in AAFD.[9] Hindfoot valgus can be better evaluated on a hindfoot alignment view radiograph by measuring the distance between the weight-bearing axis of the tibia and the most inferior aspect of the calcaneus, which has been defined as the hindfoot moment arm (Fig. 1).[10]

The abduction deformity has been measured by multiple methods in the literature and is used to divide stage II PTTD into stages IIA and IIB (Fig. 2).[1,11] Patients with less than 30% talonavicular uncoverage are classified as group IIA whereas those with greater than or equal to 30% uncoverage are classified as group IIB.[1] Other measures of midfoot abduction include the talar–first metatarsal angle and the incongruency angle.[11] The incongruency angle is formed by the intersection of a line between the lateral extent of the articular surfaces of the navicular and talus and a line between the lateral aspect of the talar neck at its most narrow segment and the lateral extent of the talar articular surface (Fig. 3).[11]

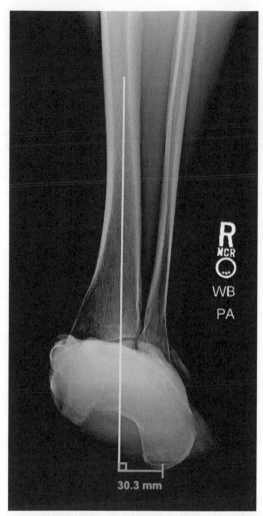

Fig. 1. Weight-bearing hindfoot alignment standard radiograph of a patient with severe hindfoot valgus. The mechanical axis of the tibia is shown in yellow. The hindfoot moment arm is shown in green, running perpendicular to the mechanical axis and measuring 30.3 mm.

Correction of the supination deformity is more difficult to assess. Measures of arch collapse, such as Meary's angle and the medial cuneiform–fifth metatarsal height, can be used as proxies for supination of the forefoot. The cuneiform articular angle (CAA), which is the angle between the proximal and distal articular surfaces of the medial cuneiform on a standing lateral radiograph of the foot, has been used to estimate the effect of a plantarflexion medial cuneiform osteotomy (Cotton osteotomy) (Fig. 4).[12]

In addition to radiographs, weight-bearing CT scans have recently been used to better characterize the deformities associated with AAFD

than traditional weight-bearing radiographs or non–weight-bearing CT scans.[9,13–17] Investigators have used weight-bearing CT scans to demonstrate that patients with AAFD have more innate talar valgus than normal control patients.[14,15] There is also a high prevalence of preoperative subfibular impingement in patients with AAFD.[16,17] Studies looking at postoperative correction of these deformities are lacking. Further research is needed to determine if increased subtalar joint valgus or severe subfibular impingement leads to inferior postoperative clinical outcomes.

Patient-reported outcomes have recently been used to evaluate the success of operative treatment of AAFD. The Foot and Ankle Outcome Score (FAOS) is 1 measurement tool that has been used and validated in AAFD.[18] The FAOS has 5 subscales, including pain, symptoms, daily activities, sports activities, and quality of life.[18] More recently PROMIS has been used in the evaluation of AAFD.[3,19] The PROMIS Physical Function, Mobility, and Pain Interference instruments demonstrated good responsiveness for AAFD with statistically significant differences between preoperative and postoperative values.[3,19] The American Orthopedic Foot & Ankle Society (AOFAS) has recently endorsed the use of the PROMIS Physical Function Computerized Adaptive Test or Lower Extremity Computerized Adaptive Test for measuring clinical outcomes for foot and ankle conditions, including AAFD.[20]

Historical Outcomes of Flatfoot Reconstruction

Initial reconstructions of adult flatfoot deformity included a medializing calcaneal osteotomy (MCO) popularized by Koutsogiannis[21] in 1971 or a lateral column lengthening (LCL) proposed by Evans in 1975.[22] Cotton[23] (1936) described an opening wedge plantarflexion osteotomy of the medial cuneiform in order to restore the tripod effect of the foot. In 1997, Pomeroy and Manoli combined a flexor digitorum longus (FDL) transfer, MCO, LCL, and heel cord lengthening to treat stage II PTTD.[24] They performed their procedure on 20 stage II flatfeet in 17 patients and had a mean follow-up time of 17.5 months with significant postoperative improvements in radiographic parameters and patient-reported outcomes.[24]

A longer-term follow-up study of the Pomeroy and Manoli (1997) surgical technique demonstrated excellent results.[24,25] At 5-year follow-up of 28 pes planovalgus feet in 26 patients treated with this reconstructive technique,

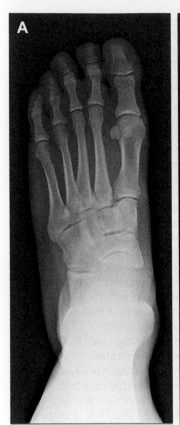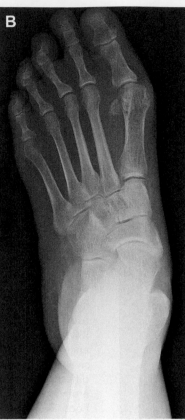

Fig. 2. (A) Weight-bearing AP standard radiographic view of the foot of a patient with stage IIA AAFD demonstrating maintenance of normal talonavicular joint alignment. (B) Weight-bearing AP standard radiographic view of the foot of a stage IIB AAFD patient demonstrating increased abduction through the talonavicular joint with uncoverage of the talar head.

the average AOFAS ankle-hindfoot scale was 90 out of 100. There were no nonunions in their cohort.[25] One patient developed symptomatic calcaneocuboid arthritis requiring joint fusion.[25] In the early 2000s, relatively few studies commented on the outcomes of flatfoot reconstructions that used both an MCO and LCL. Bolt and colleagues[26] (2007) directly compared MCO and LCL for the reconstruction of stage IIB PTTD. They reviewed the outcomes of 42 consecutive flatfeet with 25 feet undergoing an LCL only and 17 feet reconstructed with an MCO only.[26] Patients in the LCL group maintained better correction over time than the patients in the MCO-only group.[26]

Outcomes Specific to the Medializing Calcaneal Osteotomy

Early outcome studies for the treatment of flexible AAFD focused on tendon transfer procedures in combination with an MCO. Multiple studies demonstrated excellent improvement in the mean AOFAS ankle/hindfoot rating scale at least 30 months after a flatfoot reconstruction, consisting of an FDL or flexor hallucis longus

(FHL) transfer and MCO.[27–30] Changes in radiographic parameters, however, such as midfoot abduction and measures of talonavicular sag, including Meary's angle after tendon transfer and MCO, are more controversial.[28–30] Guyton and colleagues[28] (2001) and Myerson and colleagues[30] (2004) found significant improvements in radiographic measures of midfoot abduction and the medial longitudinal arch whereas Sammarco and Hockenbury[29] (2001) found no change in Meary's angle and calcaneal pitch postoperatively. Niki and colleagues[31] (2012) reviewed 8 radiographic parameters of foot alignment preoperatively and multiple time points postoperatively after an FDL transfer and MCO. They found that only changes in the Meary's and tibiocalcaneal angle were statistically significant and maintained at 1-year follow-up.[31] The investigators also demonstrated that radiographic parameters were unlikely to change after 3 months postoperatively.[31]

None of these studies examined whether there was an appropriate amount of medialization of the calcaneal tuberosity segment. Despite limited evidence, 10 mm of intraoperative medial

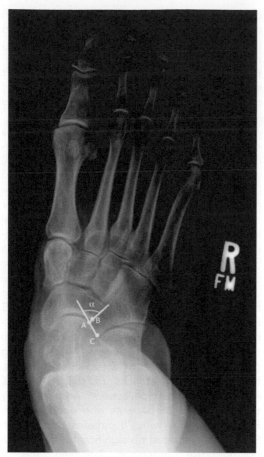

Fig. 3. The incongruency angle (α) is formed by the intersection of a line between the lateral extent of the articular surfaces of the talus (A) and navicular (B) and a line between the lateral aspect of the talar neck at its most narrow segment (C) and the lateral extent of the talar articular surface (A).

displacement of the calcaneus was frequently cited.[26,30,32–37] A biomechanical study using cadaveric feet demonstrated that a 1-cm heel slide shifted the weight distribution in the forefoot from the first and second metatarsals to the third through fifth metatarsals, which better replicates the forces in a normal foot.[38] In order to investigate the effect of the MCO on postoperative hindfoot position, Chan and colleagues[39] (2013) correlated the amount of intraoperative MCO with the change hindfoot moment arm. They found that for each millimeter of intraoperative medial heel slide, the hindfoot moment arm changed by approximately 1.5 mm between preoperative and postoperative radiographs.[39]

Conti and colleagues[40] (2015) demonstrated that a postoperative hindfoot moment arm between 0 mm and 5 mm in varus, or a clinically straight heel, led to the largest improvement in

patient-reported outcomes in the pain and symptoms FAOS subscales (**Fig. 5**). This was the first study to support an individualized amount of intraoperative MCO based on a patient's preoperative deformity. By measuring the preoperative hindfoot moment arm and using the equation proposed by Chan and colleagues[39] (2013), surgeons can theoretically preoperatively estimate the amount of intraoperative heel slide necessary.[40] Ultimately, the MCO has been shown to significantly improve clinical outcomes in patients with flexible AAFD, and the amount of MCO should be individualized for each flatfoot based on the preoperative deformity.

Outcomes Specific to Correction of Forefoot Abduction

The LCL is typically used in the treatment of patients with stage IIB PTTD in order to correct the abduction deformity at the talonavicular joint.[1] Using a 1-cm LCL graft, Sangeorzan and colleagues[41] (1993) found an average improvement in the anteroposterior (AP) talar–first metatarsal angle of 15.8° and mean correction of 26° in the talonavicular coverage angle. LCL failure, defined as either a nonunion or loss of correction, was reported to be 16.7% in 1 study.[42] There was no difference in failure rates between allograft and autograft, but the investigators did note that larger grafts were more prone to failure.[42]

Despite excellent improvement in the midfoot abduction deformity and low failure rate, the LCL puts patients at risk of lateral foot pain.[43,44] In a study comparing 10 patients who had lateral foot pain after an LCL as part of a reconstruction for stage II PTTD with 10 patients who had no lateral foot pain after LCL, the patients with lateral foot pain had increased plantar pressures on the lateral aspect of the midfoot.[44] This suggests that the addition of an LCL to a flatfoot reconstruction has the potential to overload the lateral metatarsals, cause plantar lateral foot pain, and affect patient-reported outcomes. The incidence of plantar lateral foot pain after LCL was reported to be 11.2% in a recent study.[43] The incidence was reduced using trial metal wedges so that the surgeon could intraoperatively assess eversion stiffness and the position of the foot.[43]

In order to understand how graft size affects postoperative radiographic parameters, 1 study retrospectively correlated the correction of midfoot abduction with the amount of LCL performed.[45] They found that the LCL was the only significant contributor to the change in

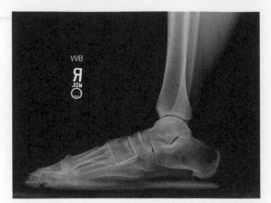

Fig. 4. Weight-bearing lateral standard radiographic view of the right foot of a patient with mild AAFD, with the CAA shown in green (0.3° plantarflexion).

the lateral incongruency angle, and, for each millimeter change in the amount of LCL, there was a 6.8° change in the lateral incongruency angle.[45] This corroborated the findings by Sangeorzan and colleagues[41] (1993) that the LCL has a significant effect on midfoot abduction.

Despite evidence that the LCL led to improvements in patient-reported outcomes, the optimal correction at the talonavicular joint had not been previously investigated.[5,24,25] A retrospective study reviewing patient-reported outcomes in 55 patients who underwent a flatfoot reconstruction for stage II PTTD found that patients corrected to a position of adduction demonstrated significantly lower improvement in the FAOS daily activities and quality-of-life subscales.[46] Adduction was defined as meeting 2 of the following 3 criteria: (1) a lateral incongruency angle less than or equal to 5°, (2) a talonavicular uncoverage angle greater than 8°, or (3) a talar–first metatarsal angle greater than 8°, which were based on previously reported radiographic measurements in this population.[11,46,47] These results suggest that

overcorrection of the talonavicular abduction deformity in patients with flexible AAFD led to inferior outcomes and should be avoided during a flatfoot reconstruction (**Fig. 6**).[46] The senior author's experience has been that using LCL graft sizes between 4 mm and 8 mm affords sufficient correction yet helps avoid overcorrection and lateral foot overload.

As an alternative to the traditional Evans opening wedge osteotomy for LCL, the step-cut lengthening calcaneal osteotomy (SLCO) was proposed was proposed by Vander Griend (2008).[48] In this technique, the anterior calcaneus is cut in a Z shape with a distal superior and vertical cut, horizontal cut, and proximal inferior and vertical cut.[48] This allows less lengthening of the lateral column and potentially a higher rate of healing because union of the osteotomy depends primarily on the horizontal aspect.[48] Clinical outcomes after an SLCO have been promising. In a cohort of 37 stage IIB PTTD patients, radiographic and patient-reported outcomes significantly improved when the SLCO was combined with an MCO.[49] Using postoperative CT scans to evaluate healing, they found no instances of delayed union, nonunion, or graft collapse.[49] Another study that compared 65 patients who underwent an Evans osteotomy with 78 patients who had an SLCO demonstrated no significant difference in postoperative outcomes between the 2 groups.[50] Patients in the SLCO group had faster healing times at the osteotomy site and fewer nonunions than the Evans group.[50] The Evans group also had larger graft sizes and a higher frequency of hardware removal than the SLCO group.[50] Consequently, the SLCO has been shown to be an acceptable alternative to the traditional Evans osteotomy for LCLs in flatfoot reconstructions, although it is technically more challenging. The dissection also requires more

A

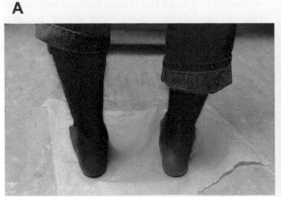

B

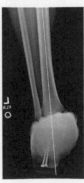

Fig. 5. (A) Clinical photo and (B) weight-bearing hindfoot alignment standard radiograph with the weight-bearing axis of the tibia shown in yellow, demonstrating neutral alignment after flatfoot reconstruction, including a 10-mm medializing posterior calcaneal osteotomy.

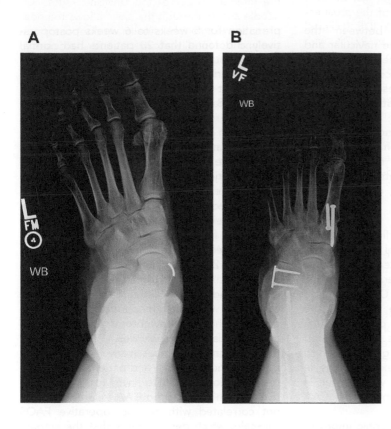

Fig. 6. (A) Weight-bearing AP standard radiographic view of the foot of a patient with stage IIB AAFD demonstrating increased midfoot abduction with uncoverage of the talar head, highlighted in yellow. (B) Weight-bearing AP standard radiographic view of the same foot after flatfoot reconstruction, including a 5-mm LCL, demonstrating optimal position of mild abduction.

lateral calcaneal stripping and dissection around the peroneal tendons.

Forefoot abduction has also been corrected by reconstructing the spring ligament using a graft passed through drill holes in the navicular and tibia or calcaneus.[51] Although there is no consensus on indications for a spring ligament reconstruction, 1 study used spring ligament reconstructions in patients with more than 30° of intraoperative talonavicular abduction or more than 10° of intraoperative talonavicular sag despite having undergone an MCO and LCL.[51] In their 13 patients who underwent spring ligament reconstructions, they found consistent improvements in clinical outcome scores and radiographic parameters of talonavicular abduction, although the investigators did not have a control group to which they could compare their results.[51]

Outcomes Specific to Correction Residual Forefoot Supination/Varus

After correction of hindfoot valgus during a flatfoot reconstruction, residual forefoot supination or varus may be present. This deformity can be addressed through a plantarflexion opening wedge osteotomy of the medial cuneiform (Cotton osteotomy) or a first TMT fusion.

Indications for a first TMT fusion include plantar-gapping at the first TMT joint, first TMT joint instability or arthritis, or a coexisting hallux valgus deformity; otherwise, a Cotton osteotomy may be used to correct the residual forefoot supination deformity.[52] Although there are few outcome studies on the use of a first TMT fusion during a flatfoot reconstruction, studies in the hallux valgus population have demonstrated excellent clinical outcomes, including return to sports and physical activity and greater than 95% union rates in patients who had complete joint preparation and rigid cross-screw fixation.[52,53]

Multiple studies have demonstrated radiographic improvement after a Cotton osteotomy as an adjunct to a flatfoot reconstruction.[54–56] In a case-control study of 67 patients who underwent a medial cuneiform opening wedge osteotomy as part of a flatfoot reconstruction and were matched with 28 control patients who did not have a Cotton osteotomy, the patients in the Cotton osteotomy group had a 6.5° statistically significant improvement in the average medial arch sag angle (MASA) compared with the control group at an average of 13 months radiographic follow-up.[56] The MASA is a measure on weight-bearing lateral radiographs of the angle between the proximal articular surface of the navicular and the distal articular surface of the medial cuneiform.[56] There was no difference, however, in Meary's angle between these 2 groups, suggesting that the Cotton osteotomy has a localized effect on midfoot sag and less of an effect on overall medial longitudinal arch height.[56] Cotton osteotomies have also been shown to have a significant effect on the CAA.[12] Postoperatively, patients, on average, had a 6.5° change in the CAA, demonstrating increased plantarflexion of the medial cuneiform.[12]

The graft size of the plantarflexion opening wedge osteotomy of the medial cuneiform has been found significantly associated with changes in CAA, calcaneal pitch, and lateral talonavicular and naviculomedial cuneiform Cobb angles.[57] When controlling for multiple variables, the only significant predictor of the change in CAA was graft size.[57] This analysis demonstrated that each millimeter increase in graft size led to a corresponding 2.1° plantarflexion change in the CAA.[57] Thus, a 4-mm graft would result in an 8.4° increase in plantarflexion of the CAA (Fig. 7).

Despite evidence for radiographic improvement in the foot after a Cotton osteotomy as part of a reconstruction for AAFD, an abstract by Vander Griend[58] (2008) suggested that residual forefoot supination could be corrected with 5 weeks to 6 weeks of postoperative casting rather through a Cotton osteotomy. After performing an MCO, medial soft tissue reconstruction, and gastrocnemius recession, he casted 28 patients with residual forefoot supination of 5° to 20° in a position of forefoot and midfoot pronation for 5 weeks to 6 weeks postoperatively and found that 20 patients had normal forefoot rotation on clinical examination and 8 patients had less than 10° of residual forefoot supination at 6 months postoperatively.[58] In a study of 63 feet in 61 patients who underwent a flatfoot reconstruction with an MCO, LCL, and Cotton osteotomy, increased postoperative CAA plantarflexion was associated with significantly lower postoperative FAOS symptoms, daily activities, sports activities, and quality-of-life subscales.[59] The size of the graft was determined intraoperatively based on the residual supination deformity after correction of hindfoot valgus and forefoot abduction.[59] When patients were divided into 2 groups, mild plantarflexion (CAA $\geq-2°$) and moderate plantarflexion (CAA $<-2°$), patients in the mild plantarflexion group had significantly better outcomes compared with the moderate plantarflexion group in the FAOS symptoms, daily activities, and sports activities subscales.[59] Preoperatively, there were no differences in any FAOS subscales between the 2 groups, and patients in the mild plantarflexion tended to have worse preoperative deformity based on CAA.[59] Graft size was not correlated with any postoperative FAOS subscale, which demonstrates that the amount of correction is less significant than final postoperative plantarflexion of the medial cuneiform.[59] This suggests that excessive plantarflexion of the medial cuneiform should be avoided when performing a Cotton osteotomy as part of a flatfoot reconstruction.[59]

Outcomes in Specific Populations

Outcome studies have also investigated the role of reconstruction of the flexible AAFD in specific

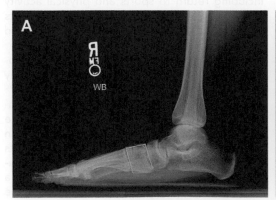
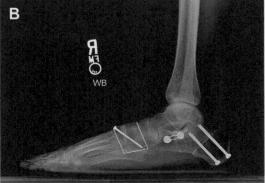

Fig. 7. (A) Weight-bearing lateral standard radiographic view of the foot of an AAFD patient with significant medial forefoot supination, with the CAA shown in green (3.1° dorsiflexion). (B) Weight-bearing lateral standard radiographic view of the same foot after flatfoot reconstruction including a 6-mm cotton osteotomy, with the CAA shown in green demonstrating resolution of the medial forefoot supination (CAA of 3.9° plantarflexion).

populations who are at higher risk of failure, including obese and older patients. Obesity is a risk factor for the development of AAFD, and the higher loads placed across the foot postoperatively puts these patients at increased risk of recollapse or nonunion of a reconstructive procedure.[60] Obese patients may also be at risk of developing wound healing complications.[61] Patients over age 65 years old also may be at risk of failing reconstruction due to less predictable healing of the osteotomies and soft tissue procedures, and some surgeons have advocated for double arthrodesis or triple arthrodesis in this group.[62] These patients may not be able to successfully navigate the recovery process or tolerate the necessary postoperative rehabilitation. Studies investigating the role of reconstruction of the flexible flatfoot in these populations have found, however, that acceptable clinical outcomes can be achieved in these groups.[61,63,64]

In a retrospective study that compared patient-reported outcomes between normal weight, overweight, and obese patients after reconstruction of the flexible AAFD, there were no differences in radiographic or clinical outcome measures, including FAOS subscales and 12-item Short Form Health Survey overall and physical component scores at 1 year postoperatively between the groups.[61] There was also no difference in postoperative complication rates; however, the study was likely underpowered to detect a difference.[61] The investigators argued that reconstruction of stage II PTTD in patients with obesity is a reasonable alternative to fusion.[61]

Another study found that reconstructions of the flexible AAFD in older patients result in clinical outcomes similar to younger patients.[63] When 140 consecutive feet were divided into groups based on age at time of surgery, patients who were 65 years old and older did not demonstrate any differences in changes in preoperative to 2 years postoperative FAOS subscales compared with younger cohorts.[63] Additionally, older patients were not more likely to undergo a subsequent revision surgery than younger patients.[63]

SUMMARY

Over the past 2 decades, flexible AAFD has been commonly treated with a combination of an FDL transfer, MCO, and heel cord lengthening with or without an LCL, Cotton osteotomy or first TMT fusion, and spring ligament reconstruction. Appropriate use of these procedures has yielded excellent clinical outcomes. Recent studies have helped to refine these procedures and attempted to provide guidelines by correlating postoperative patient-reported outcomes with radiographic measurements. The current literature suggests

- With regard to the MCO, the surgeon should aim for a clinically straight heel with a hindfoot moment arm in 0 mm to 5 mm of varus on postoperative weight-bearing hindfoot alignment view radiographs.
- When using an LCL, the talonavicular abduction deformity should not be overcorrected into a position of adduction because this may lead to inferior postoperative patient-reported outcomes.
- Excessive plantarflexion of the medial cuneiform should be avoided when performing a Cotton osteotomy as part of a flatfoot reconstruction.
- Reconstruction of the flexible AAFD is an alternative to arthrodesis in potentially high-risk populations, including obese patients and older patients over the age of 65 years old.

Further research using newer technology, such as weight-bearing CT scans, to explore how current reconstructive techniques affect the flexible flatfoot will continue to improve understanding of AAFD and should ultimately lead to better clinical outcomes.

REFERENCES

1. Deland JT. Adult-acquired flatfoot deformity. J Am Acad Orthop Surg 2008;16(7):399–406.
2. Kohls-Gatzoulis J, Woods B, Angel JC, et al. The prevalence of symptomatic posterior tibialis tendon dysfunction in women over the age of 40 in England. Foot Ankle Surg 2009;15(2):75–81.
3. Hunt KJ, Alexander I, Baumhauer J, et al. The Orthopaedic Foot and Ankle Outcomes Research (OFAR) network. Foot Ankle Int 2014;35(9):847–54.
4. Ellis SJ. Determining the talus orientation and deformity of planovalgus feet using weightbearing multiplanar axial imaging. Foot Ankle Int 2012;33(5):444–9.
5. Deland JT, Page A, Sung I-H, et al. Posterior tibial tendon insufficiency results at different stages. HSS J 2006;2(2):157–60.
6. Hiller L, Pinney SJ. Surgical treatment of acquired flatfoot deformity: what is the state of practice among academic foot and ankle surgeons in 2002? Foot Ankle Int 2003;24(9):701–5.

7. McCormick JJ, Johnson JE. Medial column procedures in the correction of adult acquired flatfoot deformity. Foot Ankle Clin 2012;17(2):283–98.

8. Barouk P, Barouk LS. Clinical diagnosis of gastrocnemius tightness. Foot Ankle Clin 2014;19(4):659–67.

9. Netto CDC, Kunas GC, Soukup D, et al. Correlation of clinical evaluation and radiographic hindfoot alignment in stage II adult-acquired flatfoot deformity. Foot Ankle Int 2018;39(7):771–9.

10. Saltzman CL, el-Khoury GY. The hindfoot alignment view. Foot Ankle Int 1995;16(9):572–6.

11. Ellis SJ, Yu JC, Williams BR, et al. New radiographic parameters assessing forefoot abduction in the adult acquired flatfoot deformity. Foot Ankle Int 2009;30(12):1168–76.

12. Castaneda D, Thordarson DB, Charlton TP. Radiographic assessment of medial cuneiform opening wedge osteotomy for flatfoot correction. Foot Ankle Int 2012;33(6):498–500.

13. de Cesar Netto C, Schon LC, Thawait GK, et al. Flexible adult acquired flatfoot deformity: comparison between weight-bearing and non-weight-bearing measurements using cone-beam computed tomography. J Bone Joint Surg Am 2017;99(18):e98.

14. Cody EA, Williamson ER, Burket JC, et al. Correlation of talar anatomy and subtalar joint alignment on weightbearing computed tomography with radiographic flatfoot parameters. Foot Ankle Int 2016;37(8):874–81.

15. Probasco W, Haleem AM, Yu J, et al. Assessment of coronal plane subtalar joint alignment in peritalar subluxation via weight-bearing multiplanar imaging. Foot Ankle Int 2015;36(3):302–9.

16. Malicky ES, Crary JL, Houghton MJ, et al. Talocalcaneal and subfibular impingement in symptomatic flatfoot in adults. J Bone Joint Surg Am 2002;84(11):2005–9.

17. Jeng CL, Rutherford T, Hull MG, et al. Assessment of bony subfibular impingement in flatfoot patients using weight-bearing CT scans. Foot Ankle Int 2019;40(2):152–8.

18. Mani SB, Brown HC, Nair P, et al. Validation of the foot and ankle outcome score in adult acquired flatfoot deformity. Foot Ankle Int 2013;34(8):1140–6.

19. Koltsov JCB, Greenfield ST, Soukup D, et al. Validation of patient-reported outcomes measurement information system computerized adaptive tests against the foot and ankle outcome score for 6 common foot and ankle pathologies. Foot Ankle Int 2017;38(8):870–8.

20. Kitaoka HB, Meeker JE, Phisitkul P, et al. AOFAS position statement regarding patient-reported outcome measures. Foot Ankle Int 2018;39(12):1389–93.

21. Koutsogiannis E. Treatment of mobile flat foot by displacement osteotomy of the calcaneus. J Bone Joint Surg Br 1971;53(1):96–100.

22. Evans D. Calcaneo-valgus deformity. J Bone Joint Surg Br 1975;57(3):270–8.

23. Cotton FJ. Foot statics and surgery. N Engl J Med 1936;214(8):353–62.

24. Pomeroy GC, Manoli A. A new operative approach for flatfoot secondary to posterior tibial tendon insufficiency: a preliminary report. Foot Ankle Int 1997;18(4):206–12.

25. Moseir-LaClair S, Pomeroy G, Manoli A. Intermediate follow-up on the double osteotomy and tendon transfer procedure for stage II posterior tibial tendon insufficiency. Foot Ankle Int 2001;22(4):283–91.

26. Bolt PM, Coy S, Toolan BC. A comparison of lateral column lengthening and medial translational osteotomy of the calcaneus for the reconstruction of adult acquired flatfoot. Foot Ankle Int 2007;28(11):1115–23.

27. Wacker JT, Hennessy MS, Saxby TS. Calcaneal osteotomy and transfer of the tendon of flexor digitorum longus for stage-II dysfunction of tibialis posterior. Three- to five-year results. J Bone Joint Surg Br 2002;84(1):54–8.

28. Guyton GP, Jeng C, Krieger LE, et al. Flexor digitorum longus transfer and medial displacement calcaneal osteotomy for posterior tibial tendon dysfunction: a middle-term clinical follow-up. Foot Ankle Int 2001;22(8):627–32.

29. Sammarco GJ, Hockenbury RT. Treatment of stage II posterior tibial tendon dysfunction with flexor hallucis longus transfer and medial displacement calcaneal osteotomy. Foot Ankle Int 2001;22(4):305–12.

30. Myerson MS, Badekas A, Schon LC. Treatment of stage II posterior tibial tendon deficiency with flexor digitorum longus tendon transfer and calcaneal osteotomy. Foot Ankle Int 2004;25(7):445–50.

31. Niki H, Hirano T, Okada H, et al. Outcome of medial displacement calcaneal osteotomy for correction of adult-acquired flatfoot. Foot Ankle Int 2012;33(11):940–6.

32. Fayazi AH, Nguyen HV, Juliano PJ. Intermediate term follow-up of calcaneal osteotomy and flexor digitorum longus transfer for treatment of posterior tibial tendon dysfunction. Foot Ankle Int 2002;23(12):1107–11.

33. Guha AR, Perera AM. Calcaneal osteotomy in the treatment of adult acquired flatfoot deformity. Foot Ankle Clin 2012;17(2):247–58.

34. Hadfield MH, Snyder JW, Liacouras PC, et al. Effects of medializing calcaneal osteotomy on Achilles tendon lengthening and plantar foot pressures. Foot Ankle Int 2003;24(7):523–9.

35. Mosier-LaClair S, Pomeroy G, Manoli A 2nd. Operative treatment of the difficult stage 2 adult acquired flatfoot deformity. Foot Ankle Clin 2001; 6(1):95–119.

36. Nyska M, Parks BG, Chu IT, et al. The contribution of the medial calcaneal osteotomy to the correction of flatfoot deformities. Foot Ankle Int 2001; 22(4):278–82.

37. Wacker J, Calder JDF, Engstrom CM, et al. MR morphometry of posterior tibialis muscle in adult acquired flat foot. Foot Ankle Int 2003;24(4):354–7.

38. Arangio GA, Salathe EP. A biomechanical analysis of posterior tibial tendon dysfunction, medial displacement calcaneal osteotomy and flexor digitorum longus transfer in adult acquired flat foot. Clin Biomech (Bristol, Avon) 2009;24(4):385–90.

39. Chan JY, Williams BR, Nair P, et al. The contribution of medializing calcaneal osteotomy on hindfoot alignment in the reconstruction of the stage II adult acquired flatfoot deformity. Foot Ankle Int 2013; 34(2):159–66.

40. Conti MS, Ellis SJ, Chan JY, et al. Optimal position of the heel following reconstruction of the stage II adult-acquired flatfoot deformity. Foot Ankle Int 2015;36(8):919–27.

41. Sangeorzan BJ, Mosca V, Jr STH. Effect of calcaneal lengthening on relationships among the hindfoot, midfoot, and forefoot. Foot Ankle Int 1993;14(3): 136–41.

42. Vosseller JT, Ellis SJ, O'Malley MJ, et al. Autograft and allograft unite similarly in lateral column lengthening for adult acquired flatfoot deformity. HSS J 2013;9(1):6–11.

43. Ellis SJ, Williams BR, Garg R, et al. Incidence of plantar lateral foot pain before and after the use of trial metal wedges in lateral column lengthening. Foot Ankle Int 2011;32(07):665–73.

44. Ellis SJ, Yu JC, Johnson AH, et al. Plantar pressures in patients with and without lateral foot pain after lateral column lengthening. J Bone Joint Surg Am 2010;92(1):81–91.

45. Chan JY, Greenfield ST, Soukup DS, et al. Contribution of lateral column lengthening to correction of forefoot abduction in Stage IIb adult acquired flatfoot deformity reconstruction. Foot Ankle Int 2015;36(12):1400–11.

46. Conti MS, Chan JY, Do HT, et al. Correlation of postoperative midfoot position with outcome following reconstruction of the Stage II adult acquired flatfoot deformity. Foot Ankle Int 2015; 36(3):239–47.

47. Kang S, Charlton TP, Thordarson DB. Lateral column length in adult flatfoot deformity. Foot Ankle Int 2013;34(3):392–7.

48. Vander Griend R. Lateral column lengthening using a "Z" osteotomy of the calcaneus. Tech Foot Ankle Surg 2008;7(4):257–63.

49. Demetracopoulos CA, Nair P, Malzberg A, et al. Outcomes of a stepcut lengthening calcaneal osteotomy for adult-acquired flatfoot deformity. Foot Ankle Int 2015;36(7):749–55.

50. Saunders SM, Ellis SJ, Demetracopoulos CA, et al. Comparative outcomes between step-cut lengthening calcaneal osteotomy vs traditional evans osteotomy for stage IIB adult-acquired flatfoot deformity. Foot Ankle Int 2018;39(1): 18–27.

51. Williams BR, Ellis SJ, Deyer TW, et al. Reconstruction of the spring ligament using a peroneus longus autograft tendon transfer. Foot Ankle Int 2010; 31(7):567–77.

52. Mani SB, Lloyd EW, MacMahon A, et al. Modified lapidus procedure with joint compression, meticulous surface preparation, and shear-strain-relieved bone graft yields low nonunion rate. HSS J 2015; 11(3):243–8.

53. MacMahon A, Karbassi J, Burket JC, et al. Return to sports and physical activities after the modified lapidus procedure for hallux valgus in young patients. Foot Ankle Int 2016;37(4):378–85.

54. Hirose CB, Johnson JE. Plantarflexion opening wedge medial cuneiform osteotomy for correction of fixed forefoot varus associated with flatfoot deformity. Foot Ankle Int 2004;25(8): 568–74.

55. Lutz M, Myerson M. Radiographic analysis of an opening wedge osteotomy of the medial cuneiform. Foot Ankle Int 2011;32(3):278–87.

56. Aiyer A, Dall GF, Shub J, et al. Radiographic correction following reconstruction of adult acquired flat foot deformity using the cotton medial cuneiform osteotomy. Foot Ankle Int 2016;37(5): 508–13.

57. Kunas GC, Do HT, Aiyer A, et al. Contribution of medial cuneiform osteotomy to correction of longitudinal arch collapse in Stage IIb adult-acquired flatfoot deformity. Foot Ankle Int 2018;39(8): 885–93.

58. Vander Griend R. Reconstruction of stage 2 posterior tibial tendon deficiency without surgical correction of residual forefoot varus. In: American Orthopaedic Foot and Ankle Society 2008 Annual Meeting. Denver, Colorado, June 26 - 28, 2008.

59. Conti MS, Garfinkel JH, Kunas GC, et al. Postoperative medial cuneiform position correlation with patient-reported outcomes following cotton osteotomy for reconstruction of the stage II adult-acquired flatfoot deformity. Foot Ankle Int 2019; 40(5):491–8.

60. Holmes GB, Mann RA. Possible epidemiological factors associated with rupture of the posterior tibial tendon. Foot Ankle 1992;13(2): 70–9.

61. Soukup DS, MacMahon A, Burket JC, et al. Effect of obesity on clinical and radiographic outcomes following reconstruction of stage II adult acquired flatfoot deformity. Foot Ankle Int 2016;37(3): 245–54.

62. Pinney SJ, Lin SS. Current concept review: acquired adult flatfoot deformity. Foot Ankle Int 2006;27(1): 66–75.

63. Conti MS, Jones MT, Savenkov O, et al. Outcomes of reconstruction of the stage II adult-acquired flatfoot deformity in older patients. Foot Ankle Int 2018;39(9):1019–27.

64. Oh I, Williams BR, Ellis SJ, et al. Reconstruction of the symptomatic idiopathic flatfoot in adolescents and young adults. Foot Ankle Int 2011;32(03): 225–32.

Peroneal Tendon Pathology
Treatment and Reconstruction of Peroneal Tears and Instability

Sophia R. Bahad[a], Justin M. Kane, MD[b,c,d,*]

KEYWORDS

- Peroneal tendon • Peroneus longus • Peroneus brevis • Peroneal retinaculum
- Peroneal instability • Lateral ankle pain • Tendon transfer • Tubularization

---

KEY POINTS

- Peroneal tendon pathology is becoming a more commonly understood source of lateral-sided ankle pain.
- Early diagnosis in peroneal tendon pathology is important in dictating treatment and ensuring optimal outcomes.
- A strong clinical suspicion coupled with physical examination findings and advanced imaging studies is necessary to accurately diagnose peroneal tendon pathology.
- The surgical treatment of peroneal tendon tears results in good to excellent outcomes with most patients returning to their preinjury level of function with positive patie nt reported outcome measures.

INTRODUCTION

One of the first reported cases of peroneal pathology was a peroneal dislocation in a ballerina by Monteggia in the 1800s.[1] Despite a body of literature replete with data, peroneal tendon instability is still often confused for lateral ligament sprains and a definitive diagnosis can be delayed in up to 40% of cases.[2] More recently, there has been an evolution in the understanding of the anatomy, mechanisms of injury, and different pathologies. Although still considered uncommon, peroneal tendon tears are recognized as a not rare cause of lateral ankle pain, especially when the pain is located posterior to the distal aspect of the fibula.

A multitude of pathologic conditions affecting the peroneal tendons can cause lateral ankle pain, including stenosing tenosynovitis, subluxation and dislocation, tendinosis, tenosynovitis, pathology related to the os peroneum,

and peroneal tendon tears. With respect to acute peroneal tendon subluxations and dislocations, conservative treatment renders recurrent instability approximately 50% of the time. Numerous investigators advocate for early surgical intervention for cases of acute peroneal tendon instability when considering the high rate of failure coupled with the typically young, active patient population.[3,4]

Comparatively, cases of symptomatic chronic peroneal tendon instability predominantly indicate for surgical intervention. Cases concerning peroneal tendon tears are categorized as either acute or chronic tears. It is important to recognize the temporal relationship of acute versus chronic is not the time to presentation. In fact, acute peroneal tears perpetually occur after a traumatic injury, yet often go unappreciated and present in a delayed manner. It is their relationship to an injury that categorizes them as

---

Disclosure Statement: The authors have nothing to disclose.
[a] The Orthopedic Institute of North Texas, PA, Baylor Frisco - Professional Building #1, 5575 Warren Parkway, #115, Frisco, TX 75034, USA; [b] Foot and Ankle Surgery Division; [c] The Orthopedic Institute of North Texas, PA, Baylor Frisco - Professional Building #1, 5575 Warren Parkway, #115, Frisco, TX 75034, USA; [d] Orthopaedics, Texas A&M University HSC, College of Medicine
* Corresponding author.
E-mail address: Justin.kane@oint.org

acute. Conversely, chronic tears tend to be attritional in nature and have an insidious onset of pain. When evaluating patients with lateral ankle pain, the clinician must maintain high suspicion of peroneal tendon pathology. With a thorough understanding of anatomy, biomechanics, the spectrum of disease states of the tendons, and several treatment options, the clinician can elect appropriate treatment algorithms to optimize the patient's recovery and return to activity. Although countless publications report high rates of success regarding several surgical treatment modalities, a dearth of high-level studies exist. Clinicians are limited in their decision-making with respect to the optimal treatment of peroneal tendon instability. Limited evidence-based data exist, with only level III and level IV studies to draw from.

ANATOMY

The lateral compartment of the lower leg includes the peroneus brevis and peroneus longus muscles and tendons. They course posterior to the fibula at the level of the ankle curve distally at the fibular tip within the retromalleolar groove. Both muscles receive their innervation from the superficial peroneal nerve and act as the primary everters of the foot. Additionally, they offer weak contribution to plantarflexion because they pass posterior to the midaxis of the tibiotalar joint.

The peroneus brevis originates at the distal two-thirds of the lateral fibula and inserts on the lateral aspect of the fifth metatarsal base. The ovoid peroneus brevis tendon courses directly posterior to the fibula, which is coated with fibrocartilage to enhance gliding. The musculotendinous junction of the brevis lies at a variable location; although typically proximal to the superior peroneal retinaculum (SPR), anatomic variation often results in a low-lying muscle belly that extends within or distal to the level of the SPR. A low-lying muscle belly is recognized as a potential cause for peroneal inflammation at the level of the SPR due to increased volume within the retrofibular space.[5]

The peroneus longus originates near the head of the fibula and upper one-half to two-thirds of the lateral fibular shaft, as well as the lateral condyle of the tibia. The peroneus longus continues plantarly through the cuboid groove before eventually inserting on the medial cuneiform and first metatarsal base. The musculotendinous junction of the peroneus longus lies proximal to that of the peroneus brevis and its tendon has a more circular morphology. With

contraction, the peroneal longus tendon compresses the brevis against the fibula. As the tendons of the peroneus brevis and longus course distally beneath the SPR, they enter the retromalleolar groove, a fibroosseous tunnel through which the peroneal tendons share a common tendon sheath approximately 2.5 to 3.5 cm from the fibular tip to the level of the peroneal tubercle. The 2 tendons then separate into their individual tendon sheaths with the brevis sitting above the peroneal tubercle and the longus below. The peroneus brevis sits closer to the fibula and glides along the fibrocartilage lining of the retromalleolar groove. A higher incidence of peroneal tendon pathology has been reported in patients whose musculotendinous junction of the peroneus brevis lies within the retromalleolar groove.[5] This is considered to be a result of the increased volume of tendon and muscle within the fibroosseous canal, which cannot expand, therefore increasing pressure on the peroneus brevis tendon against the distal fibula.[6]

The retromalleolar groove's morphology was described in a study by Edwards.[7] Of cadaveric specimens, 82% were concave, ranging from slight concavity to 3-mm depth, 11% had a flat retromalleolar groove, and 7% were convex. In most patients, the sulcus of the retromalleolar groove was 6 to 7 mm wide. A 3-mm to 4-cm long lip of fibrocartilaginous tissue borders the retromalleolar groove, therefore increasing stability of the tendons in a similar manner to the labrum in the glenohumeral articulation.[8] The medial border of the groove is formed with the posterior talofibular ligament, calcaneofibular ligament (CFL), and the posterior-inferior tibiofibular ligaments. Although it was previously postulated that a flat or convex peroneal groove played a role in peroneal tendon stability, a study by Adachi and colleagues[9] found no correlation between the retromalleolar morphology and rate of peroneal dislocations.

The SPR forms the posterior and lateral borders of the retromalleolar groove. Several studies have identified the SPR as the primary restraint to peroneal instability.[6-10] Davis and colleagues[11] conducted a cadaveric study to assess the anatomy of the SPR. All specimens shared a common origin along the periosteum of the posterolateral ridge of the fibula. The width of the footprint of the origin demonstrated a higher degree of variation. A total of 5 distinct insertions were reported. The os peroneum, a sesamoid bone within the peroneus longus near the cuboid groove, has varying degrees of ossification and is reported to exist in nearly

20% of patients in anatomic studies.[12] It is key to identify the os peroneum as a plausible pain generator. Painful fractures of the os peroneum have a high correlation with peroneus longus tears but are often overlooked.

Both muscles receive their blood supply from the peroneal artery. Petersen and colleagues[13] performed a cadaveric study to better understand the blood supply to the tendons. Near the fibular tip, the peroneus brevis has a single avascular zone as the tendon approaches its insertion. Two avascular zones were recognized in the peroneus longus. The first present as the tendon spans from the distal tip of the fibula to the peroneal tubercle, and the second while coursing through the cuboid notch. This sequence of avascularity is coherent because it correlates to frequent areas of tendonpathy.

The peroneus quartus muscle is an anatomic variant present within the lateral compartment of the leg in up to 21.7% of patients. It typically originates from the peroneus brevis muscle belly and inserts on the peroneal tubercle of the lateral calcaneus. It is thought to result in attenuation of the SPR and hypertrophy of the peroneal tubercle. Similar to the low-lying muscle belly, attenuation of the SPR is thought to result from the increased volume within the fibroosseous tunnel when the peroneus quartus muscle is present. Both the hypertrophy of the peroneal tubercle and the peroneus quartus tendon can lead to stenosing synovitis.[14]

BIOMECHANICS

Physiologic hindfoot valgus is vital for properly functioning balance of the peroneal tendons. With excessive valgus hindfoot alignment, the tendons are constricted between the fibular tip and lateral calcaneus, which may cause subfibular impingement and tendinosis. A varus hindfoot alignment may increase strain on the peroneal tendons, therefore making the patient susceptible to a spectrum of peroneal pathology.

The peroneal tendons act as the primary everters of the foot, with 63% of eversion strength attributed to the peroneal tendons, the peroneus brevis is accountable for 28%, and the peroneus longus is accountable for the other 35%.[15] These 2 tendons counterbalance the tibialis posterior and tibialis anterior. Not only do the peroneal tendons evert the foot but they also contribute 4% to plantarflexion as they span posterior to the midaxis of the tibiotalar joint in the sagittal plane. Furthermore, dynamic stability of the ankle greatly relies on the peroneal tendons.

Mann[16] described the function of the peroneal tendons using the gait cycle. The tendons are active during the stance phase of gait in which they begin firing at 12% of the cycle. At midstance, while the foot rests flat on the floor, the tendons fire eccentrically. Then, at heel rise, the tendons start to contract concentrically. Immediately before toe-off, they become quiescent at 50% of the gait cycle.

INCIDENCE AND ETIOLOGIC FACTORS
Peroneal Instability
Traumatic subluxation and dislocation of the peroneal tendons has invariably been reported with sports-related activities, especially those that involve extensive lateral movement.[17–19] Several studies have shown the SPR to be the primary restraint to dislocation of the peroneal tendons.[8,17] Forceful contraction of the peroneal tendons within the retromalleolar groove produces sufficient energy to disrupt the SPR either by tearing through its periosteal attachment on the fibula or by vigorous subperiosteal elevation. Both mechanisms permit the tendons to dislocate or subluxate.[10,17,20–22]

Debate exists as to which position of the foot is most likely to cause subluxation or dislocation. The foot positioned in dorsiflexion and eversion with a forceful contraction of the peroneal tendons is most frequently described.[23] This position allows the peroneal tendons to contract an anterolaterally directed force, therefore overcoming the SPR's restraint.[24]

Other studies suggest that acute peroneal tendon instability can be attributed to a forceful contraction with an inverted position of the foot.[25] The CFL is strained with the foot dorsiflexed and inverted, thus limiting the space within the retromalleolar groove. This reduced space causes a forceful contraction of the peroneal tendons, contributing to the likelihood of tearing of the SPR and subluxating or dislocating.[22,26] For this reason, it is hypothesized that peroneal tendon instability has a correlation to lateral ankle instability. Two separate cadaveric studies demonstrated the peroneal tendons as secondary stabilizers of the lateral ankle, with sectioning of the lateral ligaments resulting in a predisposition to injury of the SPR, resulting in peroneal tendon instability.[27,28]

Peroneal Tendon Tears
Acute tears prove to be less common than chronic tears and require severe clinical suspicion to accurately diagnose. Sammarco[29] reported that even with acute onset of symptoms, only 1 patient was diagnosed within

2 weeks of sustaining a traumatic inversion injury. On average, the duration of symptoms persisted approximately 7 to 48 months before accurate diagnosis. Arbab and colleagues[30] similarly described the relative delay in diagnosis with acute peroneal tears, considering that an accurate diagnosis was made nearly 11 months after the onset of symptoms during a study. The predominant theme, including in other studies that exist mainly in case report formats, is that in cases of acute tendon ruptures, an antecedent inversion type ankle injury occurred and the longus tendon was disproportionately affected.[31–33]

The general incidence of both acute and chronic peroneal tendon tears is considered significantly more common than previously postulated. In a cadaveric study, Sobel and colleagues[34] found a 37% (21 out of 57) incidence of peroneus brevis tears, with the majority existing within the retrofibular groove. They concluded that mechanical trauma was a probable cause for tearing, considering their location.

Sammarco and DiRaimondo[35] reported that 23% (11 out of 47) of patients experienced concomitant pathology in a study evaluating the incidence of peroneus brevis pathology in patients facing lateral ligament stabilization. DiGiovanni and colleagues[36] observed the incidence of peroneal pathology in patients treated surgically for chronic lateral ankle instability. Attenuation of the SRP was noted in 54% of patients, tenosynovitis was noted in 77% of patients, and peroneus tears were noted in 25% of patients.

A radiographic study by O'Neil and colleagues[37] examined 294 MRIs in which no hindfoot pathology was surmised, and identified some evidence of peroneal pathology in 35% (103 out of 294), despite a lack of symptoms or antecedent injury.

Several studies have attempted to identify the actual incidence of tendon involvement when pathology of the peroneal tendons exists. Peroneus brevis tears in 88% of patients surgically treated for peroneal pathology were reported in a study by Dombek and colleagues. Only 13% of patients experienced peroneus longus tears, whereas 38% of patients had concomitant tears of both tendons.[38,39]

Although most peroneus brevis tears occur in the retromalleolar groove, peroneus longus tears have 2 discrete patterns of tearing. When tearing was present at the cuboid notch, 100% were complete tears. Of patients with tears proximal to the peroneal tubercle, 8 out of 9 had partial tears. Moreover, a higher proclivity for concomitant peroneus brevis tears was found when the peroneus longus tendon had been affected at the cuboid notch.[40]

Thompson and Patterson[41] noted the strikingly reduced frequency of peroneus longus tears compared with brevis tears, which tend to occur after a trauma or sports-related injury. Kilkelly and McHale[42] further examined the role of sports-related injuries on peroneus longus ruptures with their description of an acute peroneus longus tear in a competitive runner.

CLASSIFICATION OF PERONEAL TENDON DISLOCATION

Seventy-three operative cases of acute peroneal tendon dislocations were originally described by Eckert and Davis.[8] Grade I dislocations involved elevation of the SPR from the fibula along with the fibular periosteum, thus permitting the tendons to displace between the fibula and periosteum. Grade II dislocations involved the elevation of the SPR, including the fibular periosteum and the fibrocartilaginous rim of tissue bordering the lateral aspect of the fibula. This allowed the tendons to displace between the periosteum and fibula. Meanwhile, grade III dislocations involved an avulsion of cortical bone from the lateral aspect of the fibula, including the fibrocartilaginous rim, the periosteum, and the SPR thus, allowing the tendons to displace between the fibula and periosteum. Grade IV dislocations were described by Oden[23] as torn SPRs that permitted the peroneal tendons to dislocate through the rent in the retinaculum.

The distinctive case of intrasheath peroneal tendon subluxation was noted by Raikin and colleagues.[43] Two distinct groups of patients were reported in cases in which the SPR remained intact while the tendons subluxated within the retromalleolar groove. Type A patient group was described as having an intrasheath subluxation involving intact tendons that shift their anatomic alignment within the retromalleolar groove with circumduction of the ankle; whereas the intrasheath subluxation of type B patient group involved a split tear in the peroneus brevis tendon through which the peroneus longus tendon herniates with circumduction of the ankle.

CLINICAL PRESENTATION

Accurately diagnosing an acute peroneal tendon tear is quite challenging. Patients presenting with an acute tear consistently sustained an inversion injury, causing lateral-sided ankle and/or hindfoot pain and swelling. Differentiating a peroneal tear from an ankle sprain proves to be difficult on initial presentation. Therefore, the clinician must be of high suspicion for peroneal pathology considering the multitude of other pathologic conditions that can cause lateral-sided ankle pain. Studies approximate that the delay in diagnosis of peroneal tears varies from 11 to 48 months, with a paucity of cases diagnosed on initial presentation.[29,30] Although diagnosing a peroneal tear acutely may not necessarily alter the patient's acute treatment, an accurate diagnosis is integral in counseling a patient with regard to their rehabilitation potential and possible need for future surgical intervention.

Step one to making an accurate diagnosis is to inspect the affected extremity. Because hindfoot varus is posited to contribute to the incidence of peroneal tendon pathology, a standing examination is vital. One study found that 82% of patients with peroneus longus pathology also presented a cavovarus alignment.[40] This study was further expounded on by Manoli and Graham[44] who reported that retrofibular swelling was as common in patients with peroneus brevis tears. Redfern and Myerson[39] noted that there is a high likelihood for peroneus brevis tears and involvement of both tendons when swelling and pain transpires adjacent to the fibular tip. Swelling at the distal base of the fifth metatarsal is more likely to denote a peroneus longus tear, especially when it extends into the cuboid notch.

Pain with palpation at the retromalleolar groove and ankle instability can signify split tearing of the peroneus brevis in patients without swelling. When swelling is absent, pain and instability may be the only symptoms.[45]

Particular physical examination exercises may aid in recognizing peroneal tendon pathology. Maneuvers such as passive inversion and plantarflexion may reproduce pain, whereas resisted eversion and dorsiflexion of the ankle may cause pain along with weakness. Typically, there is weakness and pain with first ray plantarflexion when a peroneus longus tear is present.

IMAGING

When imaging patients suspected of having peroneal tendon tears, the first step is to obtain weight-bearing anteroposterior, oblique, and lateral radiographs of both the foot and ankle. It is recommended to examine plain films for common fractures associated with inversion injuries, including fractures of the malleoli, lateral talar process, and anterior process of the calcaneus and fifth metatarsal base. Avulsion from the lateral aspect of the distal fibula may be a fleck sign, thus signifying a rupture of the peroneal retinaculum.

Although soft tissue injuries such as tendon tears typically cannot be seen on radiographs, certain radiographic findings can suggest a tendon rupture. Numerous studies have described the migration of the os peroneum or diastasis of a bipartite of peroneum as a definitive sign of a peroneus longus rupture.[42,46,47] In a study by Stockton and Brodsky,[48] 87.5% of surgically confirmed cases of peroneus longus ruptures displayed radiographic evidence of a fracture or proximal migration of the os peroneum. Though not a pathognomonic sign of peroneus brevis tearing, styloid process fractures at the fifth metatarsal base have been associated with brevis tears.[49]

The ideal modality for assessing soft tissue lesions is MRI. On T2-weighted imaging, acute peroneal tears have increased signal intensity and may appear as bisected, C-shaped, or flattened.[50] A study by Khoury and colleagues[51] noted peroneus longus tears as presenting a linear or round area of increased signal intensity within the tendon on T2-weighted imaging. Bony edema, visible fractures, and diastasis of the os peroneum also serve as evidence of a peroneus longus tear.[48]

Fig. 1 demonstrates an axial T1-weighted image of the ankle at the level of the tibial plafond. The peroneus brevis is noted to be flattened with the tubular-appearing peroneus longus posterior in orientation. **Fig. 2** demonstrates an axial T1-weighted image of the ankle at the level of the peroneal tubercle. The peroneus brevis is noted to have a complete split tear, with the tubular-appearing peroneus longus between the 2 segments of the peroneus brevis.

Despite being the ideal modality for assessing soft tissue, technical challenges with MRI exist when evaluating for peroneal tendon tears. As a result of their course, the peroneal tendons are susceptible to the so-called magic angle effect, a magnetic phenomenon occurring when the tendon is positioned 55° to the axis of the magnetic field. This angular orientation increases signal intensity, which may be misdiagnosed as pathology.[52] An oblique orientation of the MRI beam toward the midfoot is suggested to potentially mitigate the magic angle effect and increase accurate diagnosis of peroneus longus tears.[53]

Stockton and Brodsky[48] reported variable diagnostic accuracy with MRI compared with

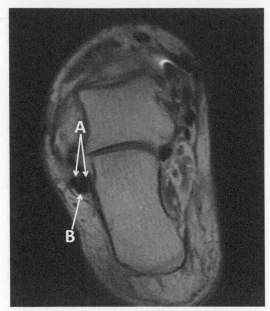

Fig. 1. Axial T1 image of the ankle at the level of the tibial plafond. The peroneus brevis (*arrows A*) is noted to be flattened with the tubular appearing peroneus longus (*arrow B*) posterior in orientation.

surgical exploration and recommended using experienced radiologists who understand the evaluated pathology. Brandes and Smith[40] recommended MRI as an advanced diagnostic

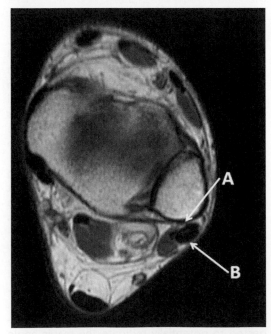

Fig. 2. Axial T1 image of the ankle at the level of the peroneal tubercle. The peroneus brevis (*arrow A*) is noted to have a complete split tear with the tubular appearing peroneus longus (*arrow B*) in between the 2 segments of the peroneus brevis.

study to ascertain the severity of peroneal tears. Counter to these studies, Redfern and Myerson[39] noted that MRI may, in fact, abate the extent of the pathology, especially with regard to peroneus longus tears. In a study concerning brevis tears, Lamm and colleagues[54] noted an 83% sensitivity and 75% specificity compared with intraoperative findings, which were expressed as flattening in MRIs of the patient in both plantarflexion and dorsiflexion. After comparing 97 MRIs to surgical results, Park and colleagues[55] concluded that MRI was specific in diagnosing peroneal tendon disorders but not sensitive. Giza and colleagues[56] attempted to correlate clinical examination with MRI findings and recorded an accurate rate of prediction with MRI to be only 48% with a high degree of incidental findings. O'Neil and colleagues[37] further confirmed these findings when they noted incidental findings indicating peroneal tendon pathology in 35% of asymptomatic patients. This discrepancy in MRI findings correlating to surgical findings should caution the clinician from solely relying on MRI for the diagnosis of peroneal tendon tears.

Under the direction of an experienced diagnostician, ultrasound can be a cost-effective, efficacious modality. Considering its relative cost compared with other advanced imaging modalities, and the lack of exposure to radiation, it can be used for diagnosis and in guiding treatment. As noted by Grant and colleagues,[57] ultrasound is 100% sensitive and 85% specific in diagnosing peroneal tendon tears. Molini and Bianchi[58] noted that ultrasound is a noninvasive, accurate dynamic modality with low morbidity in which radiation exposure is absent. Muir and colleagues[59] examined the accuracy of peroneal tendon sheath injection and concluded that ultrasound is 100% accurate for intrasheath injection. In a recent study by Framm and colleagues[60] of clinical outcomes after ultrasound-guided injection, greater than a third of patients experienced at least 3 months of pain relief with a complication rate of only 1.8%.

TREATMENT

There is an array of treatment protocols among practitioners when treating peroneal tendon tears. Treatment protocols vary greatly due to the paucity of high-quality studies pertaining to an optimal treatment algorithm. After querying foot and ankle surgeons on their management of acute peroneal tendon tears, Grice and colleagues[61] noted the distinct differences in treatment protocols and surgical techniques. Of the surgeons in the study, 22% elected a nonoperative treatment for more than a year, whereas 33% eschewed any nonoperative interventions. When operative intervention was elected, 88% of surgeons tubularized tendons after repair, 22% extracted the peroneal tubercle if hypertrophied, and 33% excised redundant tissue. An array of different suture materials and postoperative rehabilitation protocols were also used. Sammarco[29] conducted a similar study which noted a clear variability in the treatment of acute tears. Selmani and colleagues[62] described poor evidence concerning the manner of repair for peroneal tendon tears.

Krause and Brodsky[63] suggested a treatment algorithm that depended on the amount of viable tendon remaining in cross-sectional diameter. They deduced that peroneus brevis tears should be primarily treated operatively. Preferably, tendons with less than 50% involvement have the frayed portion excised, with the remaining healthy tendon tubularized, whereas tendons with greater than 50% involvement undergo en bloc excision of the diseased tendon, with tenodesis to the other tendon.

Alternatively, Redfern and Myerson proposed a treatment algorithm which categorized tears into three patterns. Type I tears were described both tendons being intact and functioning. The torn section of the tendon could be excised and tubularized. Type II tears consisted of one torn and irreparable tendon with the other still functional. The irreparable section of the tendon should be excised in these cases. Lastly, type III tears were described as neither tendon being functional. In these cases, a tendon transfer serves as the optimal treatment.[39]

In cases of irreparable tendons, allograft intercalary tendon reconstruction has been proposed. Pellegrini and colleagues[64] used a cadaveric model testing strength of loading in the tendons of the foot and ankle. In a comparison between tenodesis and allograft reconstruction, allograft tension more closely replicated that of normal tendon tension. Newer clinical evidence is being published on this technique but high level evidence is lacking with respect to its long term efficacy.

Fig. 3 demonstrates the intraoperative image corresponding to the MRI from **Fig. 1**. After intraoperative evaluation, the midsubstance of the peroneus brevis tendon was found to be unsalvageable (see **Fig. 3A**). The decision was made to perform a peroneus longus to peroneus brevis transfer. 2 to 0 nonabsorbable suture was used to perform a side-to-side tenodesis of the viable proximal and distal segments of the peroneus brevis to the intact peroneus longus (see **Fig. 3B**).

Fig. 4 demonstrates the intraoperative image corresponding to the MRI from **Fig. 2**. Evaluation of the peroneus brevis tendon was found to have significant flattening (see **Fig. 4A**). After evaluating the tendon, the decision was made to perform a tubularization procedure with excision of the nonviable portion of the tendon (see **Fig. 4B**).

OUTCOMES

Although there is a lack of evidence in the current body of literature in regards to the outcomes after the surgical management of peroneal tendon pathology, many of the studies report favorable outcomes with respect to patients returning to the activities they enjoy and their preinjury level of function.

Most the studies report relatively successful outcomes regarding surgically treated peroneal tendon tears. Accurately diagnosing patients with peroneal tendon tears is necessary to ensure successful and predictable outcomes.[30]

Krause and Brodsky[63] reported a 95% satisfaction rate with a mean postoperative AOFAS

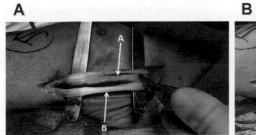
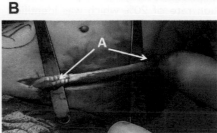

Fig. 3. (*A*) Peroneus brevis tear intraoperatively. The peroneus brevis (*arrow A*) is oriented superior to the peroneus longus (*arrow B*). (*B*) The area of nonsalvageable peroneus brevis has been excised and there has been a side-to-side tenodesis (*arrows A*) of the proximal and distal stumps of the peroneus brevis to the intact peroneus longus.

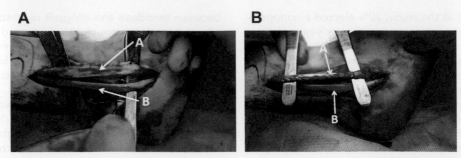

Fig. 4. (A) Significant peroneus brevis tendinosis with flattening intraoperatively. The peroneus brevis (*arrow A*) is oriented superior to the peroneus longus (*arrow B*). (B) The area tendinosis at the midsubstance of the peroneus brevis (*arrow A*) has been debrided and a tubularization has been performed. The intact peroneus longus (*arrow B*) is posterior to the peroneus brevis tubularization.

score of 85 (54–100) after the surgical management of peroneal tendon tears. Redfern and Myerson[39] obtained similar results in a study with 91% of patients achieving normal to moderate peroneal strength and a mean postoperative American Orthopedic Foot and Ankle Society Score (AOFAS) score of 82. They concluded that peroneus brevis tears performed better surgically than longus tears. Another study reported 87% of patients partaking in sporting-activities within an average of 3.5 months and a mean postoperative AOFAS score of 91.[65] Demetracopoulos and colleagues[66] described the long-term results on primary repairs of peroneal tendon tears, noting the drastic decrease in visual analog scale scores from 39 preoperatively to 10 at the time of final follow-up (*P*<.001), with a marked increase in lower extremity function score from 45 preoperatively to 71 at the time of final follow-up (*P*<.001). Only 1 patient was unable to fully return to sporting-activities.

According to a retrospective review of surgically treated peroneal tendon tears conducted by Dombek and colleagues,[2] 98% of patients experienced no limitations or pain at final follow-up; however, they did report a minor complication rate of 20% which was identified as transient symptomatology. The incidence of major complications, meaning chronic symptoms or a need for additional surgery, was reported at 10%.

A study concerning surgical treatment of all peroneal pathologies, excluding subluxation, reported the mean time to return to work as 2.5 months, whereas the mean time to return to sporting-activities was 8.5 months. Approximately 94.1% of patients were either satisfied or very satisfied with the outcomes of their procedure.[67]

SUMMARY

Though previously considered uncommon, high clinical suspicion coupled with a profound understanding of anatomy and pathophysiology of lateral ankle injuries has led to early diagnosis and treatment, thus directly improving outcomes of injuries to the peroneal tendons.

REFERENCES

1. Monteggia GB. Instituzioni chirurgiche, part III. Milan (Italy): Stamperia Pirottae Maspero; 1803. p. 336–41.
2. Dombek MF, Lamm BM, Saltrick K, et al. Peroneal tendon tears: a retrospective review. J Foot Ankle Surg 2003;42:250–8.
3. Earle AS, Moritz JR, Trapper EM. Dislocation of the peroneal tendons at the ankle: an analysis of 25 ski injuries. Northwest Med 1972;71:108–10.
4. Poll RG, Duijfues F. Treatment of recurrent dislocation of peroneal tendons. J Bone Joint Surg 1984; 66B:98–100.
5. Roster B, Michelier P, Giza E. Peroneal tendon disorders. Clin Sports Med 2015;34(4):525–641.
6. Geller J, Lin S, Cordas D, et al. Relationship of a low-lying muscle belly to tears of the peroneus brevis tendon. Am J Orthop 2003;32:541–4.
7. Edwards ME. Relations of peroneal tendons to fibula, calcaneus, and cuboideum. Am J Anat 1928;42: 213–53.
8. Eckert WR, Davis EA Jr. Acute rupture of the peroneal retinaculum. J Bone Joint Surg 1976;58A:670–3.
9. Adachi N, Fukuhara K, Kobayashi T, et al. Morphologic variations of the fibular malleolar groove with recurrent dislocation of the peroneal tendons. Foot Ankle Int 2009;30(6):540–4.
10. Niemi WJ, Savidakis J Jr, DeJesus JM. Peroneal subluxation: a comprehensive review of the literature with case presentations. J Foot Ankle Surg 1997;36:141–5.

11. Davis WH, Sobel M, Deland J, et al. The superior peroneal retinaculum: an anatomic study. Foot Ankle Int 1994;15:271–5.

12. Sobel M, Pavlov H, Geppert MJ, et al. Painful os peroneum, syndrome: a spectrum of conditions responsible for plantar lateral foot pain. Foot Ankle Int 1994;15(3):112–24.

13. Petersen W, Bobka T, Stein V, et al. Blood supply of the peroneal tendons. Injection and immunohistochemical studies of cadaver tendons. Acta Orthop Scand 2000;71:168–74.

14. Sobel M, Levy ME, Bohne WH. Congenital variations of the peroneus quartus muscle: an anatomic study. Foot Ankle Int 1990;11:81–9.

15. Clark HD, Kitaoka HB, Ehman RL. Peroneal tendon injuries. Foot Ankle Int 1998;19(5):280–8.

16. Mann RA. Overview of the foot and ankle biomechanics. In: Jahss MD, Melvin H, editors. Disorders of the foot and ankle: medical and surgical management. 2nd edition. Philadelphia: WB Saunders; 1991. p. 385–408.

17. Arrowsmith SR, Fleming LL, Allman FL. Traumatic dislocations of the peroneal tendons. Am J Sports Med 1983;11:142–6.

18. Clanton TO, Schon LC. Athletic injuries to the soft tissues of the foot and ankle. In: Mann RA, Coughlin MJ, editors. Surgery of the foot and ankle. Sixth edition. St Louis (MO): CV Mosby Co; 1993. p. 1095–224.

19. Sarmiento A, Wolf M. Subulxation of the peroneal tendons. Case treated by rerouting tendons under the calcaneofibular ligament. J Bone Joint Surg 1975;57A:115–6.

20. Martens MA, Noyez JF, Mulier JC. Recurrent dislocation of the peroneal tendons: Results of rerouting the tendons under the calcaneofibular ligament. Am J Sports Med 1986;14:114–50.

21. Marti R. Dislocation of the peroneal tendons. Am J Sports Med 1977;5:19–22.

22. Stover CN, Brytan DR. Traumatic dislocation of the peroneal tendons. Am J Surg 1962;103:180–6.

23. Oden RR. Tendon injuries about the ankle resulting from skiing. Clin Orthop Relat Res 1987;216:63–9.

24. Mason RB, Henderson JP. Traumatic peroneal tendon instability. Am J Sports Med 1996;24:652–8.

25. Safran MR, O'Malley D Jr, Fu FH. Peroneal tendon subluxation in athletes: new exam technique, case reports, and review. Med Sci Sports Exerc 1999;31(7 Suppl):S487–92.

26. Zoellner G, Clancy W Jr. Recurrent dislocation of the peroneal tendon. J Bone Joint Surg Am 1979;61:292–4.

27. Sobel M, Warren RF, Brourman S. Lateral ankle instability associated with dislocation of the peroneal tendons treated by the Chrisman-Snook procedure. A case report and literature review. Am J Sports Med 1990;18:539–43.

28. Geppert MJ, Sobel M, Bohne WH. Lateral ankle instability as a cause of superior peroneal retinacular laxity: an anatomic and biomechanical study of cadaveric feet. Foot Ankle 1993;14:330–4.

29. Sammarco GJ. Peroneus longus tendon tears: acute and chronic. Foot Ankle Int 1995;16(5):245–53.

30. Arbab D, Tingart M, Frank D, et al. Treatment of isolated peroneus longus tears and a review of the literature. Foot Ankle Spec 2014;7(2):113–8.

31. Abraham E, Stirnaman JE. Neglected rupture of the peroneal tendons causing recurrent sprains of the ankle. Case Report. J Bone Joint Surg Am 1979;61(8):1247–8.

32. Davies JA. Peroneal compartment syndrome secondary to rupture of the peroneus longus. A case report. J Bone Joint Surg Am 1979;61(5):783–4.

33. Evans JD. Subcutaneous rupture of the tendon of peroneus longus. Report of a case. J Bone Joint Surg Br 1966;48(3):507–9.

34. Sobel M, DiCarlo EF, Bohne WH, et al. Longitudinal splitting of the peroneus brevis tendon: an anatomic and histologic study of cadaveric material. Foot Ankle 1991;12(3):165–70.

35. Sammarco GJ, DiRaimondo CV. Chronic peroneus brevis tendon lesions. Foot Ankle 1989;9(4):163–70.

36. DiGiovanni BF, Fraga CJ, Cohen BE, et al. Associated injuries found in chronic lateral ankle instability. Foot Ankle Int 2000;21(1):809–15.

37. O'Neil JT, Pedowitz DI, Kerbel YE, et al. Peroneal tendon abnormalities on routine magnetic resonance imaging of the foot and ankle. Foot Ankle Int 2016;37(7):743–7.

38. Slater HK. Acute peroneal tendon tears. Foot Ankle Clin 2007;12(4):659–74.

39. Redfern D, Myerson M. The management of concomitant tears of the peroneus longus and brevis tendons. Foot Ankle Int 2004;25:695–707.

40. Brandes CB, Smith RW. Characterization of patients with primary longus tendinopathy: a review of twenty-two cases. Foot Ankle Int 2000;21(6):462–8.

41. Thompson FM, Patterson AH. Rupture of the peroneus longus tendon. Report of three cases. J Bone Joint Surg Am 1989;71(2):293–5.

42. Kilkelly FX, McHale KAS. Acute rupture of the peroneal longus tendon in a runner: a case report and review of the literature. Foot Ankle Int 1994;15:567–9.

43. Raikin SM, Elias I, Nazarian LN. Intrasheath subluxation of the peroneal tendons. J Bone Joint Surg Am 2008;90:992–9.

44. Manoli A 2nd, Graham B. The subtle cavus foot, "the underpronator". Foot Ankle Int 2005;26(3):256–63.

45. Bonnin M, Tavernier T, Bouysset M. Split lesions of the peroneus brevis tendon in chronic ankle laxity. Am J Sports Med 1997;25(5):699–703.

46. Bianchi S, Abdelwahab IF, Tegaldo G. Fracture and posterior dislocation of the os peroneum associated with rupture of the peroneus longus tendon. Can Assoc Radiol J 1991;42(5):340–4.

47. Tehranadeh J, Stoll DA, Gabriele OM. Case report 271. Posterior migration of the os peroneum of the left foot, indicating a tear of the peroneal tendon. Skeletal Radiol 1984;12(1):44–7.

48. Stockton KG, Brodsky JW. Peroneus longus tears associated with pathology of the os peroneum. Foot Ankle Int 2014;35(4):346–52.

49. Brigido MK, Fessell DP, Jacobson JA, et al. Radiography and US of os peroneum fractures and associated peroneal tendon injuries: initial experience. Radiology 2005;237:235–41.

50. Major NM, Helms CA, Fritz RC, et al. The MR imaging appearance of longitudinal split tears of the peroneus brevis tendon. Foot Ankle Int 2000;21:514–9.

51. Khoury NJ, el-Khoury GY, Saltzman CL, et al. Peroneus longus and brevis tendon tears: MR imaging evaluation. Radiology 1996;200:833–41.

52. Erickson SJ, Prost RW, Timins ME. The "magic angle" effect: background physics and clinical relevance. Radiology 1993;188(1):23–5.

53. Rademaker J, Rosenberg ZS, Delfaut EM, et al. Tears of the peroneus longus tendon: MR imaging features in nine patients. Radiology 2000;214:700–4.

54. Lamm BM, Myers DT, Dombek M, et al. Magnetic resonance imaging and surgical correlation of peroneus brevis tears. J Foot Ankle Surg 2004;43:30–6.

55. Park HJ, Lee SY, Park NH, et al. Accuracy of MR findings in characterizing peroneal tendon disorders in comparison with surgery. Acta Radiol 2012;53:795–801.

56. Giza E, Mak W, Wong SE, et al. A clinical and radiological study of peroneal tendon pathology. Foot Ankle Spec 2013;6(6):417–21.

57. Grant TH, Kelikian AS, Jereb SE, et al. Ultra-sound diagnosis of peroneal tendon tears. A surgical correlation. J Bone Joint Surg Am 2005;87:1788–94.

58. Molini L, Bianchi S. US in peroneal tendon tear. J Ultrasound 2014;17(2):125–34.

59. Muir JJ, Curtiss HM, Hollman J, et al. The accuracy of ultrasound-guided and palpation-guided peroneal tendon sheath injections. Am J Phys Med Rehabil 2011;90(7):564–71.

60. Framm BR, Rogero R, Fuchs D, et al. Clinical outcomes and complications of peroneal tendon sheath ultrasound-guided cortisone injection. Foot Ankle Int 2019;40(8):888–94.

61. Grice J, Watura C, Elliot R. Audit of foot and ankle surgeons' management of acute peroneal tendon tears and review of management protocols. Foot (Edinb) 2016;26:1–3.

62. Selmani E, Gjata V, Gjika E. Current concepts review: peroneal tendon disorders. Foot Ankle Int 2006;27(3):221–8.

63. Krause JO, Brodsky JW. Peroneus brevis tendon tears: pathophysiology, surgical reconstruction, and clinical results. Foot Ankle Int 1998;19(5):271–9.

64. Pellegrini MJ, Glisson RR, Matsumoto T, et al. Effectiveness of allograft reconstruction vs tenodesis for irreparable peroneus brevis tears: a cadaveric model. Foot Ankle Int 2016;37(8):803–8.

65. Saxena A, Cassidy A. Peroneal tendon injuries: an evaluation of 49 tears in 41 patients. J Foot Ankle Surg 2003;42:215–20.

66. Demetracopoulos CA, Vineyard JC, Kiesau CD, et al. Long-term results of debridement and primary repair of peroneal tendon tears. Foot Ankle Int 2014;35(3):252–7.

67. Grasset W, Mercier N, Chaussard C, et al. The surgical treatment of peroneal tendinopathy (excluding subluxations): a series of 17 patients. J Foot Ankle Surg 2012;51(1):13–9.

Moving?

Make sure your subscription moves with you!

To notify us of your new address, find your **Clinics Account Number** (located on your mailing label above your name), and contact customer service at:

Email: journalscustomerservice-usa@elsevier.com

800-654-2452 (subscribers in the U.S. & Canada)
314-447-8871 (subscribers outside of the U.S. & Canada)

Fax number: 314-447-8029

Elsevier Health Sciences Division
Subscription Customer Service
3251 Riverport Lane
Maryland Heights, MO 63043

*To ensure uninterrupted delivery of your subscription, please notify us at least 4 weeks in advance of move.

Printed and bound by CPI Group (UK) Ltd, Croydon, CR0 4YY

03/10/2024

01040374-0019